# Death, Dying, and Bereavement:
## Providing Compassion During a Time of Need

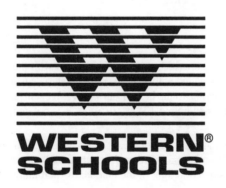

By
**Barbara Rubel, BS, MA, CBS, BCETS**

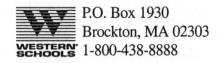

P.O. Box 1930
Brockton, MA 02303
1-800-438-8888

## ABOUT THE AUTHOR

**Barbara Rubel, BS, MA, CBS, BCETS,** Director of the Griefwork Center, Inc. in Kendall Park, NJ, is the author of *But I Didn't Say Goodbye: For Parents and Professionals Helping Child Suicide Survivors.* Rubel was featured in the 1998 PBS Emmy winning documentary, *Fatal Mistakes: Families Shattered by Suicide.* Barbara Rubel serves as a consultant for the Department of Justice Office for Victims of Crime. She travels across the U.S. offering training on issues related to traumatic grief, sudden loss and compassion fatigue in health care professionals. Barbara is an Adjunct in the Health and Nutrition Sciences Department at Brooklyn College. Rubel received her BS in Psychology and her MA in Community Health with Thanatology concentration and is a Certified Bereavement Specialist, Certified Pastoral Bereavement Counselor, and has a Certificate of Advanced Study in the Skilled Helper on the issues of Complicated Mourning. Rubel is a Board Certified Expert in Traumatic Stress and Diplomate, American Academy of Experts in Traumatic Stress, and she is a member of the Association for Death Education and Counseling.

## ABOUT THE SUBJECT MATTER REVIEWER

**Dr. Charlotte Stephenson** is professor and academic coordinator at Mississippi College School of Nursing. She has been involved in nursing education for over 25 years, and has specialized in maternal-child health. She has a BS degree in nursing, MS degree in maternal-child health nursing, and a Masters in Religious Education. Her doctorate is in Maternal-Child Health nursing with emphasis on care of the high-risk neonate and family. In her role in nursing education, she has worked to integrate caring for the dying across the life span within the nursing curriculum. She has made presentations on death and dying and end-of-life issues to nurses and other health care providers. She has participated in the End-of-Life Nursing Education Consortium sponsored by the American Associate of Colleges of Nursing and the City of Hope.

**Nurse Planner:** Amy Bernard, RN, BSN, MS

**Copy Editor:** Demi Rasmussen

**Indexer:** Sylvia Coates

**ISBN:** 1-57801-107-8

# IMPORTANT: Read these instructions *BEFORE* proceeding!

Enclosed with your course book, you will find the FasTrax® answer sheet. Use this form to answer all the final exam questions that appear in this course book. If you are completing more than one course, be sure to write your answers on the appropriate answer sheet. Full instructions and complete grading details are printed on the FasTrax instruction sheet, also enclosed with your order. Please review them before starting. *If you are mailing your answer sheet(s) to Western Schools, we recommend you make a copy as a backup.*

## ABOUT THIS COURSE

A Pretest is provided with each course to test your current knowledge base regarding the subject matter contained within this course. Your Final Exam is a multiple choice examination. **You will find the exam questions at the end of each chapter.**

In the event the course has less than 100 questions, leave the remaining answer boxes on the FasTrax answer sheet blank. **Use a <u>black</u> pen to fill in your answer sheet.**

## A PASSING SCORE

You must score 70% or better in order to pass this course and receive your Certificate of Completion. Should you fail to achieve the required score, we will send you an additional FasTrax answer sheet so that you may make a second attempt to pass the course. Western Schools will allow you three chances to pass the same course...*at no extra charge!* After three failed attempts to pass the same course, your file will be closed.

## RECORDING YOUR HOURS

Please monitor the time it takes to complete this course using the handy log sheet on the other side of this page. See below for transferring study hours to the course evaluation.

## COURSE EVALUATIONS

In this course book, you will find a short evaluation about the course you are soon to complete. This information is vital to providing Western Schools with feedback on this course. The course evaluation answer section is in the lower right hand corner of the FasTrax answer sheet marked "Evaluation," with answers marked 1–16. Your answers are important to us; please take a few minutes to complete the evaluation.

On the back of the FasTrax instruction sheet, there is additional space to make any comments about the course, the school, and suggested new curriculum. Please mail the FasTrax instruction sheet, with your comments, back to Western Schools in the envelope provided with your course order.

## TRANSFERRING STUDY TIME

Upon completion of the course, transfer the total study time from your log sheet to question 16 in the course evaluation. The answers will be in ranges; please choose the proper hour range that best represents your study time. You **MUST** log your study time under question 16 on the course evaluation.

## EXTENSIONS

You have two (2) years from the date of enrollment to complete this course. A six (6) month extension may be purchased. If after 30 months from the original enrollment date you do not complete the course, *your file will be closed and no certificate can be issued.*

## CHANGE OF ADDRESS?

In the event you have moved during the completion of this course, please call our student services department at 1-800-618-1670, and we will update your file.

## A GUARANTEE TO WHICH YOU'LL GIVE HIGH HONORS

If any continuing education course fails to meet your expectations or if you are not satisfied in any manner, for any reason, you may return it for an exchange or a refund (less shipping and handling) within 30 days. Software, video, and audio courses must be returned unopened.

*Thank you for enrolling at Western Schools!*

WESTERN SCHOOLS
P.O. Box 1930
Brockton, MA 02303
(800) 438-8888
www.westernschools.com

# Death, Dying and Bereavement:
## Providing Compassion During a Time of Need

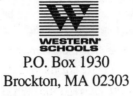

P.O. Box 1930
Brockton, MA 02303

Please use this log to total the number of hours you spend reading the text and taking the final examination (use 50-min hours).

| Date | Hours Spent |
|------|-------------|
| _____ | _____ |
| _____ | _____ |
| _____ | _____ |
| _____ | _____ |
| _____ | _____ |
| _____ | _____ |
| _____ | _____ |
| _____ | _____ |
| _____ | _____ |
| _____ | _____ |
| _____ | _____ |
| _____ | _____ |
| _____ | _____ |

TOTAL ☐

**Please log your study hours with submission of your final exam. To log your study time, fill in the appropriate circle under question 16 of the FasTrax® answer sheet under the Evaluation section.**

# Death, Dying and Bereavement:
## Providing Compassion During a Time of Need

### WESTERN SCHOOLS
### CONTINUING EDUCATION EVALUATION

Instructions: Mark your answers to the following questions with a black pen on the Evaluation section of your FasTrax® answer sheet provided with this course. You should not return this sheet.

Please use the scale below to rate how well the course content met the educational objectives.

|   |   |   |   |
|---|---|---|---|
| A | Agree Strongly | C | Disagree Somewhat |
| B | Agree Somewhat | D | Disagree Strongly |

After completing this course I am able to

1. introduce the historical perspective of death, attitudes toward death, and the contemporary American death system.

2. distinguish factors that influence the grief process and identified the differences between bereavement and mourning.

3. identify the types of suicide, some risk factors for suicide, and the differences between suicide prevention, intervention, and postvention.

4. characterize ways individuals cope with life-threatening illness and dying, focusing on how to provide support to those who are dying and exploring the issues facing the family of the dying patient.

5. report on advance directives and issues facing family members and individuals at the end of life.

6. describe the dimensions of anticipatory mourning, the reactions of family members after the death of their loved one, grief interventions, effective communication techniques before, during, and after the death, and interventions for death notification.

7. illustrate life span issues facing grieving children, adolescents, adults, and the elderly.

8. identify various means of bereavement support.

9. characterize ways to prevent burnout and compassion fatigue and described particularly difficult end-of-life situations.

10. The content of this course was relevant to the objectives.

11. This offering met my professional education needs.

12. The objectives met the overall purpose/goal of the course.

13. The course was generally well-written and the subject matter explained thoroughly. (If no, please explain on the back of the FasTrax instruction sheet.)

14. The content of this course was appropriate for home study.

15. The final examination was well-written and at an appropriate level for the content of the course.

16. **PLEASE LOG YOUR STUDY HOURS WITH SUBMISSION OF YOUR FINAL EXAM.**
    Please choose which best represents the total study hours it took to complete this 30-hour course.

    A. less than 25 hours        C.  29–32 hours

    B. 25–28 hours               D.  greater than 32 hours

# CONTENTS

# FIGURES & TABLES

# PRETEST

1. Begin this course by taking the Pretest. Circle the answers to the questions on this page, or write the answers on a separate sheet of paper. Do not log answers to the Pretest questions on the FasTrax test sheet included with the course.

2. Compare your answers to the PRETEST KEY located in the back of the book. The Pretest answer key indicates the course chapter where the content of that question is discussed. Make note of the questions you missed, so that you can focus on those areas as you complete the course.

3. Complete the course by reading each chapter and completing the exam questions at the end of the chapter. Answers to these exam questions should be logged on the FasTrax test sheet included with the course.

1. The three most common causes of death for those 65 years old and over in the United States are

   a. chronic lower respiratory disease, influenza, and pneumonia.

   b. diabetes, Alzheimer's disease, nephritis.

   c. diseases of the heart, accidents, and septicemia.

   d. diseases of the heart, malignant neoplasms, and cardiovascular disease.

2. Burial, cremation, entombment, and body donation are associated with

   a. final disposition.

   b. final arrangements.

   c. embalming.

   d. entombment.

3. The type of funeral where a celebrant facilitates the funeral by meeting with family and friends of the deceased, listens to their stories, takes notes, and then creates a shared picture including the relationships with those who attend is known as

   a. cremation.

   b. fun.

   c. traditional.

   d. secular, life-centered.

4. Regressive behaviors may cause those who grieve to

   a. return to a behavior from an earlier time in life.

   b. become sexually promiscuous.

   c. increase drug use.

   d. talk non-stop.

5. The customs, beliefs, values, and attitudes that are shared by a specific group of people is known as

   a. mourning.

   b. bereavement.

   c. culture.

   d. grief.

6. The number of elderly persons who complete suicide every 1 hour 39.3 minutes is

   a. one.
   b. three.
   c. six.
   d. nine.

7. The most common method of suicide in the United States is

   a. drowning.
   b. carbon monoxide poisoning.
   c. hanging.
   d. firearms.

8. The type of denial where patients accept the terminal diagnosis but still talk as if they will survive is

   a. denial of facts.
   b. denial of implications.
   c. denial of extinction.
   d. death denial.

9. An open-ended question used to identify the patient's perspective on his or her illness is

   a. "Do you think that you will get better?"
   b. "Do you think your family is keeping anything from you?"
   c. "Have you talked with any other dying patients?"
   d. "How are you coping with all this?"

10. According to Rando, a conflicting demand of anticipatory grief is

    a. planning for life before the death of the loved one versus not wanting to betray the loved one by considering life in his or her absence.
    b. letting go of the ill person versus moving on.
    c. experiencing the full intensity of feelings involved in anticipatory mourning versus trying to avoid becoming relaxed.
    d. acknowledging the terrible reality and its implications versus trying to maintain some hope.

11. To improve the quality of time spent with a dying patient or with a family member who is experiencing either anticipatory mourning or bereavement, you should

    a. be more willing just to be there, without doing anything.
    b. ignore awareness of your energy levels to avoid exhaustion and burnout.
    c. impose your philosophy of dying on the person you are seeking to help.
    d. be dishonest with yourself about what you are willing to give to the dying or bereaved.

12. A specific service provided to grieving family members immediately after a death in a hospital is to

    a. call a chaplain, minister, rabbi, or priest whether or not the family wants spiritual support.
    b. discard all belongings of the deceased.
    c. offer bereavement therapy.
    d. make immediately available at the time of loss a secluded, quiet, nicely furnished room as a place for family privacy.

13. When a family member has died at home, children are least likely to not to want to go into the room where the death occurred if they are

    a. between the ages of 1 and 3.

    b. between the ages of 3 and 5.

    c. between the ages of 5 and 8.

    d. between the ages of 8 and 11.

14. The understanding that death is inevitable to living things and that all living things die reflects the concept of

    a. personal mortality.

    b. irreversibility.

    c. universality.

    d. causality.

15. The understanding that death is final and that, once dead, a person cannot become alive again is called

    a. non-functionality.

    b. irreversibility.

    c. universality.

    d. causality.

16. Children who understand the universality of death, that not only do "all living things die" but that "I will die," have reached an understanding of

    a. non-functionality.

    b. causality.

    c. irreversibility.

    d. personal mortality.

17. The sorrow one feels over the loss of a loved one can last

    a. 6 months.

    b. 1 year.

    c. 10 years.

    d. a lifetime.

18. Grieving people can be helped in support groups by

    a. discussing the changes in their lives since the death.

    b. controlling their feelings in the presence of others.

    c. encouraging unforgiveness.

    d. keeping personal stories private and focusing on others.

19. The caring awareness of another person's anguish and, at the same time, a need to lessen it is

    a. burnout.

    b. bereavement.

    c. compassion.

    d. mourning.

20. Whether health professionals experience grief or avoid it, their grieving process is influenced by their

    a. private experiences with loss.

    b. personal loss histories and work style.

    c. individual differences.

    d. ability to withdraw.

# INTRODUCTION

This continuing education course is designed to provide fundamental knowledge about death, dying, and bereavement. The major premise of this book is that every health professional can learn ways to support those who are dying, those who companion them, and those who mourn their death. This course is intended to be a key resource for nurses and nursing home administrators who are called upon in loss situations. By taking this course, you may develop an overall understanding of death studies, including the grief process; suicide and life-threatening behavior; caring for the dying; life span issues for children, adolescents, adults, and the elderly; how to help the bereaved cope with loss; and professional caregiver issues.

Beginning with a basic understanding of death education and the changing encounters of death through the years, the course reviews the contemporary American death system. Palliative care nurses will learn how they can provide support to those who are dying and develop an understanding of what they and their families are experiencing. After taking this course, nurses will be able to describe palliative care, hospice principles, and the significance of the stage-based and task-based models for coping with death and dying. ED nurses are frequently called upon in sudden loss situations. Whether a perinatal, child, teenager, adult, or elderly death, nurses will learn ways to provide immediate support to grieving family members and identify ways to help them cope. Nurses will become skilled at how to deliver bad news and understand what the survivors and victims are experiencing in order to provide compassionate care. Labor and delivery nurses will be given tools to support parents who have experienced a perinatal loss. Geriatric Nurses, who provide older adults with high quality care, will benefit from the section on life span issues. Geriatric nurses will identify the most common and difficult adjustments for grieving older adults. This course book will provide nephrology nurses with tools to use with their patient's and their family members. Nephrology nurses care for patients of all ages who are experiencing, or are at risk for, kidney disease. Bonds are formed between the patient, nurse, and family member as patients can know their nurses for years. Various modalities of therapy may require the nurse to remain with the patient for several hours. During this time, patients not only share information about their condition, but discuss their feelings and fears. Nephrology nurses will recognize meaningful communication skills that can be used with their patients during their time together. Oncology nurses will learn the significance of bereavement counseling and support groups. By becoming aware of a bereavement support network on the Internet and in their own community, they will be better able to provide immediate assistance in a time of need.

Improving the standard of patient care begins with education. Whether a radiological nurse who has been working in the field for several years or a student nurse who wants to learn about compassionate care, this course book is for them. This book will provide the education that addresses personal and professional losses and growth as nurses learn valuable ways to prevent burnout and compassion fatigue. The stages of burnout and the risk factors will be reviewed. This course book will give all nurses the opportunity to look at the strain between their satisfaction in their role in providing compassionate care and the compassion fatigue they may be experiencing.

There are personal insight boxes throughout the chapters of this course. These boxes provide the opportunity to reflect on personal issues and beliefs. The goal of this book is to familiarize nurses with death, dying, and bereavement. However, personal concerns play a role in how nurses respond to patients and family members. This book is meant not only to give professionals insight on ways to help a dying patient and family members cope but also to provide a guide and opportunity to examine personal and professional attitudes about loss.

Upon completion of this course, health care professionals will be able to demonstrate an overall understanding of thanatology, a term derived from the name of a Greek god of death. It is a discipline concerned with death and dying. The book is intended to be a practical guide to help nurses and nursing home administrators think about death and understand their feelings about the deaths of their patients. When the course is completed, nurses should have a basic knowledge of death, dying, and bereavement, applicable to any branch of nursing.

# CHAPTER 1

# DEATH STUDIES

## CHAPTER OBJECTIVE

After completing this chapter, the reader will be able to discuss the historical perspective of death, attitudes toward death, and the contemporary American death system.

## LEARNING OBJECTIVES

After studying the material in this chapter, the reader will be able to

1. specify three ways that death education is conducted in the United States.

2. identify common euphemisms that replace the words "death," "dead," and "dying."

3. identify seven death categories.

4. indicate five components of the contemporary American death system.

## THANATOLOGY

*"Cry woe, destruction, ruin, loss, decay:*
*The worst is death, and death will have his day."*
— Shakespeare

Thanatology, a term derived from Thanatos, the name of the Greek god of death, is a discipline concerned with death and dying. Health professionals, due to the very nature of their work, may come in contact with those who are dying or grieving. They may also be called upon to offer assistance to their own family members who are experiencing loss. Individuals equate nursing with compassionate care giving and so family members may rely more on a nurse in the family than someone from another profession. Most nurses are periodically involved to some extent in thanatology. At one time or another nurses are likely to be involved in providing treatment to those who are dying, tending to those who have just died, or offering support to those who mourn them. Nurses are better able to provide this type of care when they are trained in death education.

### Death Education

Corr, Nabe, and Corr (2000) note that death education is conducted through formal education, informal education, and teachable moments.

- Formal education is usually associated with programs of organized instruction such as elementary and secondary education, college and university curricula, professional and postgraduate education, training and in-service programs for care providers, workshops, presentations, or support groups, both private and public.

- Informal education typically begins at an earlier point in time. It may start in the arms of a parent or guardian and proceed through interactions within social groups (i.e., travel, media).

- Teachable moments stem from unanticipated events in life that offer possibilities for developing useful educational insights as well as lessons for personal growth, like finding a dead bird (p. 9).

> **Personal Insight**
>
> *Are you taking this course because of a previous or ongoing personal experience?*
>
> *Are you taking this because of your involvement with dying patients?*
>
> *What do you wish to understand better concerning death, dying, and bereavement?*

Death possesses many meanings. Whether nurses learn about death education through formal or informal education or teachable moments, their experience with patients is their greatest teacher. Pfaadt (2000) notes that skilled nursing services encompass four major areas:

    a.  observation and assessment,

    b.  teaching and training,

    c.  performance of skilled treatments and pro cedures (also known as direct, hands-on care), and

    d.  management and evaluation of a client care plan (p. 297).

While managing the patient's care plan, nurses observe, assess, teach, and provide hands-on care. Through the experience of caring, nurses may be faced with situations that are complicated and emotionally draining. Skilled nursing can be enhanced by continuing nurses' education on death, dying, and bereavement. Examples include a hospice nurse who enrolls in a workshop on palliative care, an NICU nurse who attends a conference on communication skills with families in the hospital setting, and an emergency room nurse who takes a college course on death and dying.

The primary reason for standards of education for nurses is to ensure that patients receive quality care. Ferrell, Coyne, and Uman (2000) examined basic nursing education in a group of 2,033 nurses and found that the vast majority of nurses reported their basic nursing education inadequate in all areas of end-of-life care. These areas included pain, end-of-life content, family caregiver needs, symptom management, grief, ethical issues, and care at time of death. Nurses who continue their education in end-of-life care become more adept in providing compassion in a time of need. Silverdale and Katz (2003) found that student's personal and interpersonal skills and abilities when responding to a dying person were enhanced due to taking a long-distance death and dying course. Results suggest that the students felt more confident in providing care to those who were dying.

> **Personal Insight**
>
> *How confident do you feel in providing care to those who are dying?*

Silverdale and Katz (2003) found that if health-care providers are more considerate of what a dying person is going through, they will be more confident in communicating with the dying person and will perceive themselves as having the skill to offer individualized care and patient autonomy. The study showed that caregivers exhibited positive attitudes after becoming aware of what the dying person was going through, learning effective ways to provide emotional care, and developing appropriate communication skills. Due to these changes in their attitudes, caregivers were able to develop meaningful relationships with their dying patients.

## Attitudes Toward Death

Our personal experiences with death are reflected in our attitudes about it. One definition of attitude is a mental position, feeling, or emotion toward a fact or state. Death-related attitudes develop in contemplation of one's own death or that of another person. Attitudes about what will happen as one dies, and attitudes about an afterlife stem from our personal experiences and discussions.

> **Personal Insight**
>
> *What does it mean to you to die? What do you think death feels like?*

## Media

Media is a form of informal education about death. Some people go an entire lifetime without seeing a dying or dead person. Others may have been present as someone was dying and or may have paid their respects at a service where there was an open casket. These experiences influence one's attitudes about death. Death affects all aspects of an individual's life. Whether or not we have actually seen someone die or have seen a dead person, we may have seen it in the movies or on television. In our society, television, film, and print media have become a significant form of exposing individuals to death.

In terms of the media, death is sometimes romanticized or violent. With television in every home, Americans are less isolated from violent death, especially when scenes of war are bought into our living rooms. Whether our pet dies, we learn of a famous person's death, or we have an accident, we are reminded of our own vulnerability and mortality. When someone close to us dies, our attitudes about death are tested. The way we express our attitude changes as our experiences in life change. Our perception of the event and the manner in which we respond to it is influenced by our attitudes.

Media can affect our attitudes and influence our behavior. The literature suggests that the presentation of AIDS in the media can affect the public's behavior. Burkholder, Harlow, and Washkwich (1999) studied stigma, HIV/AIDS knowledge, and sexual risk in 481 sexually active heterosexual late adolescents. The study suggests that individuals make judgments about risks to themselves based on their own personal experience and the media's portrayal of that risk. AIDS in the media can influence attitudes by educating the public about their own risk for AIDS.

Another study on the association between media presentation and influences was performed by Elasmar, Hasegawa, and Brain (1999). They investigated the portrayal of women in U.S. prime time television during the 1992-93 season, exploring the association between the way women were portrayed on television and the perception of women as important members of society outside the home. They found that the hair color of female TV characters favors the notion that blond hair is associated with attractiveness. The results indicated that the public's attitude would be influenced by the color of the character's hair. From something as simple as hair color, we can see that the media's portrayal of certain images has a direct relation to how the public views that image.

People who have not experienced a death may derive their images of death from those in television shows or movies. Media plays a significant role in presenting death, dying, and bereavement stories. By presenting these stories in an authentic and compassionate manner, public attitudes may be more positive and less death anxiety will be experienced.

> ### *Personal Insight*
> *What role do you think media has played in your attitudes about death?*

## Fear of Death

Throughout life, there are teachable moments when we learn about death. Such moments may include pointing to a dead bird on the side of a road while riding in a car with one's parents and then discussing what happened to the bird. Knowledge of death may come through informal education, as when a child sits in his mother's lap while she gently informs him that his grandmother has died after a long illness. We learn from these experiences, and our understanding of loss stems from what we saw, who we were with, and how they responded to our feelings, our questions, and most of all, our fears.

For people on the road of death, there is no turning around. All life's hopes may be gone. The mission, goals, and careers that bring value into our lives may feel meaningless. Death is the ultimate loss. The fears associated with letting go of earthly affairs and caring for those we love can contribute to death anxiety. Fear of being in pain or dying alone is shadowed by fear or uncertainty about the future. For some, there is the fear that they may go to hell. Physically, we will become non-existent, no longer having any control. Fears of pain and suffering, fears of the unknown, and concerns about the death of significant others are multiple dimensions of uncertainty.

> *Personal Insight*
> *Have you thought about what happens to your body after death? Do you envision your body being eaten by worms in the ground or being burned into ash? When you think of your own death do you experience any sense of apprehension?*

In 1933, Franklin Roosevelt said, "The only thing we have to fear is fear itself." We can avoid thinking about death in order not to face our fear. However, it is an illusion to think that we can shield ourselves from it in total. Early Egypt defied the idea that death would be the finality of life. As a death-defying society, pyramids were constructed to house not only bodies but also possessions to be brought into the next life, thus creating an illusion of control and continuity. As we face death now, we understand the influence it has in tearing down our impressions of predictability, control, and continuity (Vickio, 2000). One cannot predict what will happen in our future. However, the way we confront death is shaped by the society in which we live.

In a death-accepting society, death is looked upon as a natural and inevitable part of life. Dying and helping those who are dying are built into the daily patterns of living (Rando, 1984). Do we need to accept death? Do we need to let go and detach ourselves from the way we see ourselves? Must we accept a spiritual connection that moves us to a spiritual place shared with others who have gone before us? As we look at acceptance, we learn about ourelves. Our religious and spiritual beliefs shape our acceptance of death.

America is a death-denying society. For the most part, Americans would rather not discuss death. Many individuals create rituals to remind themselves of a death though death itself is difficult to accept. The prevalent American attitude is that death is not a normal part of human existence and opposes life (Rando, 1984). Whether we decide to keep a dying loved one at home or use a nursing home is influenced by our attitudes. Our attitudes are reflected in the fear we feel when watching someone die. Some of the ways we can express our fear about death are using defensive humor, displacing the fear onto sex or work, becoming a death-related professional, writing about death, or expressing feelings creatively through art and music (Kalish, 1985).

Our attitudes about death have a direct bearing on the decisions we make about end-of-life wishes. Men express a stronger preference for life-sustaining treatment than women depending on their current health. Women express a greater desire to have a dignified death than men. Women may not want to live with diminished cognitive and social abilities, so they often choose not to have life-sustaining treatment (Bookwala et al., 2001). Our attitudes also have a direct bearing on our approach to helping. If health professionals fear death, their opinions, beliefs, and feelings will be reflected in their attitudes about helping those who are dying and those who grieve.

Our attitudes about death stem from our experiences with loss, from our formal and informal death education training, and from teachable moments we have experienced. We develop educational insight and personal growth from teachable moments. Within those moments, we reflect upon our beliefs, and those beliefs are shown in our attitudes. Would you believe a patient who informs you they had a near-death experience (NDE)? Near-death experience occurs sometimes when the pulse and breathing has stopped. Those who have a NDE believe that they are going to die. There is a perceived threat of death. However, the individual lives through it, is resuscitated, and survives. Though no two NDE's are the same, there are similar patterns in their occurrence such as moving through a dark tunnel, experiencing intense emotions that range from happiness to anguish, and seeing a light or a deceased loved one. Those who go through a NDE may have a life review and re-experience a milestone from their past. The individual's perception of that re-experience helps them to make changes in their life.

> *Personal Insight*
> *Based on your death education and fear of death, do you believe that it is possible to sustain a near-death experience? Explain.*

Many people inform their nurse that they had a NDE during surgery, when they were physically ill, or when they had an accident. They see their bodies from a different position, whether standing next to or hovering above the body. They may have come close to death or have been clinically dead, but they recovered. The individual may feel fear, anxiety, joy, or peace.

Nurses practicing in critical care settings may come across a patient who has experienced a NDE. Whether or not the nurse believes that the NDE happened, acknowledging what the patient went through and what it means to them enhances communication. These experiences are life-altering, but many keep them secret for fear of ridicule. Those who experience a NDE may have a renewed will to live and a stronger religious faith. Nurses who are uncomfortable addressing the NDE can at least address what it means to the person that experienced it.

> *Personal Insight*
> *If you were to undergo a near-death experience, do you think you would feel terror and anger? Would your thoughts be resigned to death? Would you pray and remain calm? As you reflect on these questions, think about your first death experience. Does that experience in any way play a part in how you are responding to the questions regarding near-death experience?*

## Relationship of First Death Experience to Current Death Attitudes

This section considers the possible relationship between the personal meaning of death and past experience. According to Cicirelli (2001), personal meanings of death "are constructed by the individual and are primarily cognitive interpretations of objects and events associated with death that are derived from the individual's experience."

> *Personal Insight*
> *When you think of your first death experience, what kind of image comes to your mind? In creating that picture, is the image disturbing or does it cause anxiety?*

Death is the final stage of life. During life, most of us have experienced the death of a loved one and that image remains with us. Our current attitudes about death stem from that past experience. Therefore, reflecting on that experience will help us be aware of our current death attitudes. If those attitude cause anxiety, professional assistance is available. As mentioned in this chapter, informal education typically begins at a younger age, with a parent or guardian. How effective a health professional will be in providing support may stem from these past experiences, including those from childhood. In a study by Knight, Elfenbein, and Capozzi (2000), it was reported that the average age related to the first recalled childhood human death experience was 9.55 years. The authors concluded that more information is needed regarding the way parents talked with us as children about death, what our parents said, and our parent's affect as they discussed it.

> *Personal Insight*
> *As a child, were you allowed to attend funerals of family members? Did your parents talk about death in your presence?*

## Review of Historical Perspective of Death

From an historical perspective, we can trace death observances of humans to prehistoric times, when people would observe special ceremonies when burying their dead. As years passed, the dead were usually buried in cemeteries outside of areas where people lived.

Historically, ancient people thought of the dead as impure; their proximity was feared and bodies were not allowed to remain inside towns. Thus, ancient cemeteries were typically located outside of towns. But earlier attitudes began to change, as Christianity became the dominant mode of thought in the West. People now wanted to be buried near the bodies of the martyrs, presumably because the martyrs' relics would protect them at the Second Coming, and basilicas began to be built in these places. So when death became a tame feature of human experience, the dead ceased to inspire fear. Living people now moved around near the dead with no anxiety, and eventually all cemeteries were located near churches (Corr, Nabe, & Corr, 2000, p. 61).

In the 1330s, an outbreak of bubonic plague took place in China, a busy trading nation. In 1347, Italian merchant ships returned from a trip to the Black Sea, which was a key link in trade with China. As the ships docked in Sicily, many on board were already dying of the plague. Within days, the disease spread throughout Sicily. By August, the plague had spread to England, where it was called "the Black Death" because of the black spots on the skin. The disease was carried, often via rats, from person to person by fleas, which went dormant until the spring of 1348, when the plague struck again. After 5 years, 25 million people had died. As there were reoccurrences of the plague through the centuries, people lived in constant fear of the plague's return. The black plague largely disappeared from Europe in the 1600s.

In the 1800s, families would bury their dead in cemeteries that resembled parks. Picnics would be shared near the stones that marked their loved one's final resting place. Photos would be taken of the deceased. These photos would be sent to family members who could not attend the funeral. During the Civil War, the role of the funeral director across the United States was very significant, as bodies of dead soldiers came home needing to be buried.

During the 1800s, people died in their homes surrounded by their families. The leading causes of death at that time were tuberculosis, pneumonia, and diarrhea. At the turn of the century, approximately 30% of all deaths were among children under the age of 5. Between 1930 and 1950, there was a shift in where people died. They no longer died in their own home surrounded by family, and instead, were brought to hospitals where they usually died alone.

As we look back on the twentieth century, we see how death is a part of our common history. A hundred years ago, the average American could expect to live for only about 50 years. Infectious diseases at the time claimed many lives. Individuals continue to die from accidents, illnesses, their own hand, and in old age. The U.S. Department of Health and Human Services (2001) has found that the life expectancy in the U.S. rose to 77.2 years in 2001. Life expectancy for men is 74.4 and 79.8 for women in the United States.

The most common causes of death for those 65 and older include, in order of prevalence, diseases of the heart, malignant neoplasms, cardiovascular disease, chronic lower respiratory disease, influenza and pneumonia, diabetes, Alzheimer's disease, nephritis, accidents, and septicemia (see Table 1-1). In other age groups, accidents, homicide, suicide, and human immunodeficiency virus (HIV) are more prominent. In children 4 years of age and younger, septicemia is a common cause of death, and Alzheimer's disease is not present (Arias & Smith, 2003).

## TABLE 1-1: TEN LEADING CAUSES OF DEATH IN THE U.S.

| | |
|---|---|
| Heart Disease | 710,760 |
| Cancer | 553,091 |
| Stroke | 167,661 |
| Chronic Lower Respiratory Disease | 122,009 |
| Accidents | 97,900 |
| Diabetes | 69,301 |
| Pneumonia/Influenza | 65,313 |
| Alzheimer's Disease | 49,558 |
| Nephritis, Nephrotic Syndrome, and Nephrosis | 37,251 |
| Septicemia | 31,224 |

*Source:* Arias, E. & Smith, B.L. (2003). Deaths: Preliminary Data for 2001. *National Vital Statistics Report, 51*(5), March 14, 2003. Available online: http://www.cdc.gov/nchs/data/nvsr/nvsr51/nvsr51_05.pdf

## Death Language

As nurses and nursing home administrators, we cannot ignore language about death, death expressions, and euphemisms. Common euphemisms include:

- resting in peace,
- bought the farm,
- pushing up daisies,
- called home,
- gone away,
- merely sleeping,
- down for the long count,
- on his last legs,
- put to sleep,
- kicked the bucket,
- number is up.

Common expressions that refer to death are:

- dead ringer,
- scared to death,
- dead serious,
- dead weight,
- talk a subject to death,
- dead ahead,
- kill the lights,
- dead as a door knob,
- dying to meet you, and
- political suicide.

Euphemisms often replace the words "death," "dead," and "dying" and appear to be a more pleasant word or phrase. However, Corr et al. (2000) note that the excessive use of euphemisms when talking about death provides a distancing from this basic life event. Nurses should become fully knowledgeable about common euphemisms and expressions. Though death no longer is a taboo subject, health care professionals still use certain terms such as "passed on" or "expired" instead of using the word "dead." Being comfortable using proper death terms benefits those who mourn. This is especially true for nurses who have the responsibility of informing a family member that their loved one has died, as shown in the following example.

### Example

Sam, a 71-year-old male patient with Alzheimer's disease, has died in a nursing home. The nursing home administrator informs the patient's son that he has died, saying, "I'm sorry to inform you that your father expired." The son asks, "Do you mean my father is dead?" Repeating the phrase, the administrator says, "He expired." Sam's son once again says, "Did he die?" The administrator says, "Yes. He expired." The son says, "My dad is not a milk carton. I hope the next time you have to inform a son that his father is dead, you are more comfortable saying it like it is."

## Death Categories

*We say indeed that the hour of death is uncertain, but when we say this we imagine that hour as situated in a vague and distant future. It never occurs to us that it has any relation to the day already begun or that*

*death could come this very afternoon,*
*which is anything but uncertain—this after-*
*noon, every hour of which is filled in*
*advance.*      — Marcel Proust (1948, p.91)

Death means different things to different people. There are various death categories, with the general definition of death being the cessation of life. However, there is no such thing as the moment of death. Death is a process that takes place over time, where the body dies cell by cell. *Cell death* is the death of individual body cells. During this process, respiration, heartbeat, and brain activity stop. *Local death* is the death of a part of the body. *Brain death* is characterized by the end of all brain activity, complete unresponsiveness, and no spontaneous breathing. The lack of brain activity is indicated by a flat EEG where the individual is in deep coma and there is no muscular movement. *Cardiac death* is the moment the heart stops beating. However, one may believe that death does not truly occur until there is an end to all vital functions, as in *functional death*. A *spiritual death* is when the soul, as defined by various religions, departs the body.

We may feel dread about total annihilation and attempt to deny that we will die. When we are confronted with death, no matter what the meaning, we realize how uncertain our own lives are. Our concerns about dying and our own death anxiety are important to understand as we explore our concerns about those in our care. Anxiety is a sense of apprehension and fear often marked by physiological signs (as sweating, tension and increased pulse), by doubt concerning the reality and nature of the threat, and by self-doubt about one's capacity to cope with it. Studies have shown that men, older adults, and those who are religious report lower death anxiety.

> *Personal Insight*
> *What does death mean to you? Do you see*
> *death as extinction or a new beginning?*

Death is a loss of being alive and all the other losses that come with it, the loss of being in control, the loss of things that are important, and most importantly the loss of one's body. As we explore the ways individuals cope with death, we address anxiety as the fearful concern or interest in death. As nurses work with dying patients, the experience can trigger their own awareness of personal losses and fears about their own death. These nurses can become overwhelmed by death anxieties. This can lead them to focus only on the physical needs of their patients and evade emotional issues, which results in emotional distancing. Nurses who have not mastered the personal fear of death may find it difficult to care for those who are dying.

## THE CONTEMPORARY AMERICAN DEATH SYSTEM

Though millions die each year, and millions more are affected by these deaths, death in America continues to be a subject that is difficult to discuss. The number of deaths in 2000 in the United States was 2,403,351 (Anderson, 2002). Kastenbaum (2001) maintains, "We may think of the death system as the interpersonal, sociophysical and symbolic network through which an individual's relationship to mortality is mediated by his or her society" (p. 66). Kastenbaum's Contemporary American Death System Model includes five components: *people, places, times, objects,* and *symbols.*

Some of the *people* who work with dying and the dead or come in contact with those dying and dead include nurses, nursing assistants, bereavement counselors, home health aides, social workers, physicians, medical examiners funeral directors, EMTs, cemetery workers, florists, police officers, clergy, life insurance salesmen, counselors, and the military. Educators who teach death and dying courses, writers, and researchers are also some of the *people* that make up the system model.

Another component of Kastenbaum's death system model is *places,* such as a funeral taking place at a cemetery. Another place involved in our death system is a hospital, where many individuals die. Whether physicians or nurses give death notification in the halls or friends and family gather around the patient's bedside, the hospital represents the last place many see their loved one alive. For others, it represents the place where they hear the news of their terminal illness and where they make frequent trips as reminders of their own mortality. This is especially true for the elderly. The older individual may have health problems that cause frequent trips to the hospital. Though they may recover from each of the numerous trips, their capacity diminishes when they do not have enough reserve or resiliency to bounce back from illness. They may ultimately welcome death, which becomes an avenue to see long-lost loved ones, go to heaven, or be free of suffering (Amella, 2003).

Another component of the death system is *times* of the year that reflect society's ways to honor the dead. Memorial Day and the Day of the Dead in Mexico are two known days that mark society's mourning. Prayers for the dead are offered throughout the year, especially on anniversaries of tragic events. A year after September 11th, communities came together to mourn those who died. This will continue to be a time of year where people recognize the anniversary of the day when thousands of people lost their lives through a terrorist attack.

*Objects* also play a role in the death system. Obituaries in local newspapers, the electric chair, tombstones, and certificate of death are objects in the death system. The U.S. standard certificate of death includes the time and cause of death. After the physician signs the certificate, it is considered a legal proof of death. Caskets are also objects that make us very much aware of death. When we look at these objects, we are immediately reminded of death.

The last component of the death system are *symbols* identified with death. The color black usually symbolizes mourning. Jewish mourners wear a torn piece of black ribbon on their lapel. Wearing dark clothes at a funeral and driving dark-colored limousines for the funeral procession are also symbolic in nature. The grim reaper, who wears a long robe and skull mask, is another symbol identified with death. A Catholic symbol identified with death is the ritual of the Sacrament of the sick and last rites for dying Catholics.

> **Personal Insight**
> *What parts of the death system have you come across in your personal and professional life?*

## Functions of the Death System

The five components of the death system perform seven functions:

1. warnings and predictions,
2. preventing death,
3. caring for the dying,
4. disposing of the dead,
5. social consolidation after death,
6. making sense of death,
7. and killing (Kastenbaum, 2001).

Nurses perform some of these functions by giving patients test results, administering medications, and providing support to family members during the dying process. After a patient's death, nurses also communicate with the family and help them cope.

### Example

Fred and Grace's daughter, Hope, was born with muscular dystrophy, a degenerative condition. Grace contacted hospice after her physician informed them that Hope was terminally ill. The whole family, Fred, Grace, and Hope's brother, Steve, were present during the initial visit with the hospice nurse, Chris. Chris was present during Hope's death and attended Hope's funeral service. She provided support to the family by calling 3 weeks after the death and also contacted the family on the anniversary of Hope's death, which brought the family much comfort.

## Final Disposition

As shown in the example, families benefit from support after their loved ones die. As support is provided to the family, the issue of managing the body arises. There are certain cultural, religious, and legal requirements that must be fulfilled when disposing of the dead. Final arrangements, final disposition, embalming, entombment, or burial are common words associated with the care of corpses. Final arrangements are associated with care and disposition of a human body and the ceremony following the death. Final disposition includes burial, cremation, entombment, or body donation. Cremation comes from the Latin word *cremo*, which means "to burn." Cremation is a process of reducing the human body to bone fragments using high heat and flame. Embalming involves preserving the body by removing the blood and replacing it with formaldehyde. Entombment is when the body is placed in an above-ground mausoleum, while burial involves placement of a body in the ground, usually in a casket or vault. Another common word associated with disposing of the dead is body donation, where the body is donated to medical science.

In the United States, most body disposal is through a burial in a cemetery. Various cultures dispose of bodies in unique ways. The Parsi people of India, once Bombay's most important community, practice the Zoroastrian rite of disposing their dead in the open air. Within the Zoroastrian religion, great emphasis is placed on death rituals, with the body bathed and clothed in a shroud. It is then placed on a specially made scaffold called a dakhma. These dakhmas are also called the Tower of Silence. Bodies either decompose naturally under the sun or are eaten by vultures. Another means of corpse disposal is a water burial, where bodies are disposed of at sea. Another common corpse disposal technique in the United States is by cremation, which is also less expensive than a burial.

Disposal of the body begins with a discussion of who will become involved in funeral planning. Funeral arrangements are made when family members in advance of mourners choose a casket and decide whether the body will be buried or cremated. Though the price for burials can be as high as $15,000, Bern-Klug, DeViney, and Ekerdt (2000) found the cost for a quarter of burials was under $4,670, while a quarter of cremations cost more than $3,047.

If the family decides to have a funeral, this tradition helps the mourners come to terms with the fact that their loved one is dead. The relationship is transformed in death. Though the physical relationship is gone, a spiritual bond continues. By placing photos and mementos at the funeral home, mourners provide support to those in grief.

Funerals are usually held from the day after the death to 4 days later. There is usually a religious ceremony at a house of worship or funeral home and a burial ceremony at the gravesite. The religious ceremony can also take place at the gravesite. In special circumstances, a memorial service may be arranged where the body is not present and the focus of the service is on the person's life, not his or her death.

The family members meet with a funeral director and decide the manner in which they want their funeral service to be carried out. Everyone, whether or not they preplan the funeral, must meet with the funeral director. During this meeting, paperwork is signed with the current date or date of death. Even if everything was preplanned, it is a state law to have a current 'General Price List' and a current 'Statement of Funeral Goods and Services.' This is done in case there is anything mourners wish to append to the funeral that was not originally set in the pre-arrangements.

Three new funeral methods—cremation, secular life-centered funerals, and celebratory "fun" funerals—are replacing traditional funerals. Gadberry (2000) found that single or divorced, wealthy, college educated individuals who do not live near their family are more apt to choose cremation. He notes that some incentives for cremation include land space, environmental issues, and costs. If during the funeral arrangements the decision is made for the body to be cremated, the family members will discuss what to do with the cremains, otherwise known as ashes. No casket is required for a cremation, as a wooden or cardboard container is used and is cremated with the body. In some states, no container or embalming is required. The family may witness the body being placed into the cremation chamber. For an average size adult, cremation takes approximately 4 hours at a temperature between 1,500° F to 2,000° F.

After the cremation is complete, all organic bone fragments, which are very brittle, as well as non-consumed metal items are "swept" into the back of the cremation chamber and into a stainless steel cooling pan. All non-consumed items are separated from the cremains. Items such as dental gold and silver are non-recoverable and are commingled in with the cremains. Remaining bone fragments, whitish to light gray in color, weighing approximately 5 pounds, are processed in a machine and then placed into a temporary or permanent urn selected by the family.

Families can choose from several options regarding what to do with the ashes. They may choose from a cremation container or rental casket for the service. Families can bury the cremains in a cemetery plot. Ashes can be buried in a cremation garden or scattered across the ocean. Another common choice is to place the cremains in an urn which can be kept in a special place.

Some religious groups include cremation as part of their funeral custom. Religions that do not allow cremation are orthodox Jewish, Islamic, Eastern Orthodox, and a few fundamentalist Christian faiths. The Catholic Church accepts cremation as long as it is not chosen for reasons that are contrary to Christian teachings. Nearly all Protestant churches allow for the urn to be present during the memorial service. Most Catholic church-

es also allow the ashes to be present during the memorial Mass.

A second nontraditional funeral is the secular, life-centered funeral. A celebrant facilitates the funeral by meeting with family and friends of the deceased and listening to their stories. The celebrant takes notes and then creates a shared picture including the relationships with those who attend the funeral.

A third nontraditional method is the "fun" funeral. Fun funerals are controversial, though they show no disrespect to the person that died or the survivors. These funerals are upbeat and celebrate the person's life. Whatever the form of the funeral, memories are shared as people gather together to pay their last respects to the person who died. Through the sharing of memories, the relationships are transformed and the bond is continued. Photographs, mementos, and tributes may solidify and maintain a transformed relationship, which brings about positive memories (Gamino, Sewell, & Easterling, 2000).

> ### *Personal Insight*
> *Would you take advantage of preplanning your funeral? If you answered yes, would you do so alone or would you bring someone with you? As you think about this question, what images come to mind?*

## Death Certificates

A death certificate is a legal record of a death. Each certificate will show the date, time, place, and cause of death. A certified copy of the death certificate is necessary for life insurance and other death benefits. It is also needed for probate, which is the process that transfers legal title of property from the estate of the individual who has died. When making arrangements, statistical information for the death certificate is reviewed. During an arrangement, the funeral director addresses how many death certificates the family will need, and the following information regarding the decedent is gathered:

- full legal name,

- date and place of birth,
- home address and telephone number,
- social security number,
- occupation if applicable, along with the company, city, and state where the decsendent worked,
- veteran's serial number if applicable,
- highest level of education,
- parent's names, including mother's maiden name,
- father and mother's birthplace, and
- marital status.

Funeral directors can only get death certificates for 6 months after the death.

Death certificates are needed for the family to settle financial affairs. Organizations requiring death certificates include:

- each financial institute,
- probate court,
- Social Security,
- each life insurance company,
- stocks, bonds, and mutual fund companies,
- the IRS and state tax agency,
- pension administrators,
- each automobile creditor or lessor, and
- organizations governing each piece of real estate owned.

If the family needs to get additional death certificates, they must contact the Health Department or Registrar. The family must provide proof of who they are in the form of an I.D. (e.g., birth certificate, marriage license, income tax return). Requests for a certified death record should include the decedent's full name, place of death, relationship to the person who is requesting the record, and the reason for requesting the record.

Family members in these cases will be asked certain questions, with the answers recorded on the death certificate. This practice was instituted after the terrorists attacked on September 11th as deceitful individuals were stealing identities of deceased individuals. A law was enacted to combat this problem.

## Final Details

After the statistical information is gathered during an arrangement, other details must be reviewed.

- Funeral home
- Place of service
- Religious preference
- Religious passage selected
- Participating organizations involved (i.e. military, lodge, etc.)
- Flag preference, if used—draped or folded
- Type of viewing: none, public, or private
- Open or closed casket at the service
- Type of casket
- Type of vault
- Cremation vs. burial
- Type of urn
- Disposition of ashes
- Music, floral, and clothing preferences
- Personal accessories to stay on the body or be returned to significant other
- Pallbearers' names
- Eulogy
- Newspaper notices and names in the paper
- Memorial park or cemetery preferred
- Type of memorial marker: upright monument, memorial plaque, other
- Preference for a graveside or memorial service
- Preference to be buried near a particular person

# SUMMARY

The chapter began with the term *thanatology* being defined and the ways death education is conducted in the United States. Nurses are better able to provide care when they are trained in death education. The primary reason for standards of education for nurses were noted. Attitudes toward death and the ways that media can affect our attitudes and influence our behavior were explored. Death anxiety and fear of death are factors that play a role in how we help those who are dying, those who grieving, and our own perception of death. There is a difference between a death-accepting society and a death-denying society. Nurses who fear death will find their opinions, beliefs, and feelings reflected in their attitudes about helping those dying and those who are grieving.

This chapter also examined beliefs about near-death experiences and whether or not the nurse believes that the NDE happened. We can enhance communication by acknowledging what the patient went through and what the experience meant to them. The chapter also highlighted the relationship of the first death experience to current death attitudes, as nurses' current attitude about death stems from past experiences.

This chapter looked at a review of historical perspectives of death and death language. Death expressions and euphemisms were discussed. Death categories and what death means to different people were noted. The death categories of cell death, local death, brain death, cardiac death, functional death, and spiritual death were defined.

Kastenbaum's Contemporary American Death System model includes five components: *people, places, times, objects,* and *symbols*. The model focuses on the five components of the death system performing seven functions: warnings and predictions; preventing death; caring for the dying; disposing of the dead; social consolidation after death; making sense of death; and killing.

Near the end of the chapter, the meeting with the funeral director and what takes place during this meeting was reviewed. Topics discussed include the manner in which a funeral service can be carried out and statistical information for the death certificate.

Final disposition was examined. Certain cultural, religious, and legal requirements that must be fulfilled when disposing of the dead were discussed. The significance of death certificates was explored.

Some people memorialize a loss through a traditional funeral. The price for burials, what is involved in funeral planning, and funeral arrangements were noted. New funeral methods, cremation, secular life-centered funerals, and celebratory "fun" funerals were described. Cremation and several options as to what families can do with the ashes were examined.

# RESOURCES

## Death Studies on the Internet

Death and Dying from About.com
dying.about.com

Funerals with Love
www.funeralswithlove.com

Jewish Funerals, Burial, and Mourning
www.jewish-funerals.org

Medline Plus Health Information
www.nlm.nih.gov/medlineplus/deathand
dying.html

Online Obituary, Funeral, Cremation, and
Cemetery Resource
www.funeralnet.com

Project on Death in America
www.soros.org/death/

Resources on Funerals from the Federal Trade
Commission
www.ftc.gov/bcp/conline/pubs/services/
funeral.htm

Thanatology Newsletter, Brooklyn College
thethanatologynewsletter.com

# EXAM QUESTIONS

## CHAPTER 1
### Questions 1-10

1. The form of death education conducted through programs of organized instruction, such as elementary and secondary education or college and university curricula, is known as

   a. formal education.
   b. informal education.
   c. teachable moments.
   d. final disposition.

2. In a death accepting society, death is looked upon as a

   a. natural and inevitable part of life.
   b. topic that should be not discussed.
   c. strong preference for life sustaining treatment.
   d. abnormal part of human existence and opposing life.

3. A common euphemism for death in the United States is

   a. "he expired."
   b. insights.
   c. mausoleum.
   d. entombment.

4. The death category that best describes the death of a part of the body is

   a. brain death.
   b. spiritual death.
   c. cell death.
   d. local death.

5. The death category that refers to the end of all brain activity, complete unresponsiveness, no spontaneous breathing, and produces a deep coma is

   a. cell death.
   b. brain death.
   c. cardiac death.
   d. spiritual death.

6. The death category that best describes when the soul, as defined by various religions, departs the body is

   a. cell death.
   b. brain death.
   c. cardiac death.
   d. spiritual death.

7. The five components of Kastenbaum's model of the death system are

   a. people, places, times, death, and healing.

   b. people, places, times, objects, and symbols.

   c. people, places, death, symbols, and preventing death.

   d. people, places, objects, healing, and symbols.

8. A function of the death system is to

   a. prevent death.

   b. cheat death.

   c. object to death.

   d. symbolize death.

9. Final arrangements are associated with

   a. preserving the body by removing the blood and replacing it with formaldehyde.

   b. care and disposition of a human body and the ceremony following the death.

   c. burial, cremation, entombment, and body donation.

   d. donating the body to medical science.

10. The name of the process of reducing the human body to bone fragments using high heat and flame is

    a. burial.

    b. secular.

    c. cremation.

    d. memorial service.

# CHAPTER 2

# GRIEF, BEREAVEMENT, AND MOURNING

## CHAPTER OBJECTIVE

After completing this chapter, the reader will be able to describe factors that influence the grief process and identify the difference between bereavement and mourning.

## LEARNING OBJECTIVES

After studying this chapter, the reader will be able to

1. indicate factors that influence the grief process.
2. distinguish between normal grief and complicated grief.
3. differentiate between bereavement and mourning.
4. identify current theories of grief and mourning.

*"Man cannot live without a continuous confidence in something indestructible within himself."*
– Franz Kafka

## THE GRIEF PROCESS

The central goal of this chapter is to convey a sense of what happens in the body, mind, and spirit of those who experience the death of a significant person in their lives. Nurses and nursing home administrators should be aware of the fundamentals of the grief process, including loss, bereavement, and mourning to better understand of what the patient, the patient's family, and significant others are going through.

Kelly (2001) notes, "Grief originates from the Anglo-Norman 'gref' and the Old French meaning hardship, suffering, displeasure, grievance, hurt, injury, and mental distress" (p. 293). By simplest definition, grief refers to a process that includes the intense physical, emotional, and spiritual suffering after a loss. A loss is a final separation. Grief is used as a term to describe the symptoms, feelings, beliefs, and thoughts as a person remembers and reflects upon the loss.

### Factors That Influence Grief

#### Physical Factors

After a death, a grieving individual may experience physical reactions, such as sensitivity to noise, changes in appetite, headaches, dry mouth, neck and shoulder pain, and tightness in the chest. Females can experience menstrual irregularities. Both men and women may experience an increase in colds and infections. Other physical factors include tiredness and exhaustion, temporary slowing of reactions, muscular aches, rashes, breathlessness, tension, and exaggeration of allergies. The bereaved may also experience bowel and bladder disturbances, feelings of hollowness in the stomach, ulcers, and nausea.

Many newly bereaved individuals experience sleep disturbances. Not being able to sleep or awakening suddenly from a deep sleep are normal responses. In time, most grieving persons return to their normal sleeping pattern. The individual may not want to go to sleep for fear of having a nightmare or a dream about their loved one. Though dreams can be comforting, they can also be heartbreaking. Upon waking, dreams make the person painfully aware that their loved one is really dead. During the dream, the deceased may attempt to tell them or teach them something. In exploring the meaning of the dream and what transpired, the bereaved may attempt to figure out what their loved one was trying to tell them. This advice can clarify a problem the bereaved was having and even help them to resolve it.

If a grieving individual is having a problem sleeping, it might be due to an underlying fear of mortality. He or she may fear that they will not wake up. If their loved one died, they recognize they, too, can die, and this fear can manifest itself in their sleeping patterns. Imagine a widow, having slept with her spouse for 65 years, faced with sleeping in a bed alone after his death. During a dream, she may see her spouse walking along a beach, his favorite pasttime. In seeing him, she is made aware that he is safe and content, but she wakes up alone.

**Emotional Factors**

Emotional factors include shock, numbness, rage, loneliness, apathy, crying, sadness, anxiety, rejection, jealousy, aggression, guilt, stress, withdrawal, fear, pining, yearning, and anger. Anger can be directed at physicians, at God, at the deceased, and themselves. Even a child experiences anger when taken from its mother. Bowlby (1982) describes protest, despair, and detachment as the three phases a child goes through when separated from mother. The protest an infant feels is comparable to the anger an adult feels when separated from a loved one because of a death. When the infant's mother is not present, the infant feels abandoned and experiences protest. A grieving adult who feels abandoned and separated from a significant person feels a similar reaction of protest. Bowlby describes

despair as "preoccupation with his missing mother…increasing hopelessness…cry monotonously or intermittently…is withdrawn and inactive, makes no demands on people in the environment, and appears to be in a state of deep mourning" (p. 27). Grieving adults also experience despair after a loved one dies and are usually preoccupied with thoughts of the departed. The human experience of loss is a lifetime journey that begins as a child and ends with death.

Though grieving individuals may be preoccupied with thoughts of the deceased, they may also find relief in their death.

- A widow is no longer the caretaker of her terminally ill husband.

- A child who was brought to his grandmother's home every day and told to play quietly can now run around and make noise.

- A daughter who moved into her parent's home to help her father care for her dying mother can now move back home with her husband.

- A neighbor with a busy schedule no longer shops for her terminally ill friend.

Individuals may find relief after the death of a loved one, as they no longer watch the person suffer. However, attempts to return to life as it was before the death can bring about guilt feelings. Though they may have provided care to their loved one, they may now reflect on the things they did not do. They may say, "If only I had..." It is not uncommon to hear "If only I had taken him to the doctor sooner;" "If only I had been to see her that morning;" "If only I had forced him to take his medication and stick to his diet." As the bereaved share their "If only" with a nurse, it is best to comfort them by listening and not attempting to make them see that it was not their fault.

A nurse who listens to a widow explain how her husband's death is all her fault does not have to attempt to make the widow see how it was not her fault. By listening to her and giving her an opportunity to voice her concerns, the nurse will provide an opportunity for the individual to test this reality. It is more effective to listen and not attempt to make the widow see why she should not feel that way or change her mind. As a nurse listens, the grieving widow is allowed to express how she feels; by doing so, she will work through her issues of responsibility.

## Cognitive Factors

After the death of a significant person in one's life, the grieving individual's mind will attempt to make sense of the experience. Those in grief may experience obsessive thinking and have dreams and nightmares. The grieving person may become absent-minded, unable to concentrate, disoriented, and confused, and overly critical of their own actions. In addition, the person may attempt to avoid reminders of the loss, may not want to think about the deceased, or may continually review the circumstances of the death.

## Psychological Factors

Psychological factors that influence grief are the survivor's personality and coping skills. How has the person coped in the past with loss, and whom did they depend upon during that time? History of mental illness and depression are psychological factors that play a role in how a person copes with the death of someone close to them. Other factors that play a role in the way a person grieves are self-esteem and relationship to the deceased. If an elderly woman who loved to cook dies after 50 years of marriage, her husband may have a difficult time preparing meals. The elderly widower may not be able to cope with the death because of the dependent nature of the relationship he shared with his wife. Factors such as age and concurrent stressors play a significant role in how an individual will cope with loss. For very young grieving children and the elderly, others may need to address who will take care of them.

## Behavioral Factors

A grieving individual may experience changes in eating habits and not eat enough food. This can cause weight changes and health problems. If the grieving person experiences insomnia and has a poor appetite, the behavior can influence social factors. Changes within a grieving person's life can bring about withdrawal from friends, family, and community. At a time when support is needed, many people retreat into the private world of grief. Though a normal response, it is during this time that persons need the most support and can become aggressive, hoard, increase their drug use, increase sexual activity, become hyperactive, or talk nonstop. Regressive behaviors may cause those who grieve to return to behavior from an earlier time in their life. This is especially true for children, who may start wetting the bed and sucking their thumb after years of not doing so.

Many grieving individuals experience searching, whereby they look for their loved one in a crowd or experience an event that reminds them of their special person. As they attempt to make sense of the loss, they may cry and experience absent-minded behavior. They may place keys in the refrigerator, not recall where they parked, and forget well-known phone numbers.

## Religious Factors

Every religion has among its doctrines a point of view regarding death. These views can range from seeing death as a punishment to viewing it as a transition to a better existence. Lester et al., (2001-2002) examined university undergraduates' beliefs about the afterlife. Some of the questions regarding feelings about life after death were "Do you believe that there is life after death?" "Do you believe that the afterlife is in a specific place?" "Is there a heaven?" "Is the afterlife the same for everyone?" "Is the afterlife affected by the timing of one's death?" and "Is there a hell? (p.125). The study found that 89% of the subjects believed in life after death. Ninety percent reported that there is a heaven and 95% reported the belief that they would be reunited with family and friends in the afterlife. A significant number of students (93%) reported that the afterlife is comforting.

**Personal Insight**

*Do you believe there is a life after death? Does that belief bring you comfort?*

## Cultural Factors

*"As for a future life, every man must judge for himself between conflicting vague possibilities."*

– Charles Darwin

As a nurse, it is advantageous to be familiar with the cultural background of the patients in your care. Culture is a way of life, for a specific group of people; it includes all of their customs, beliefs, values, and attitudes. Though some health professionals may make generalizations based on their own past experiences and backgrounds, it is important to look at the grieving individual as part of a group. These groups have certain cultures, and during difficult times individuals will turn to their culture for comfort and support. Though some of their traditions may seem strange, a person's cultural beliefs help the person cope with death, dying, and bereavement.

People from around the world and from a spectrum of religious faiths are likely to be among those who nurses will help as they cope with grief. A nurse should gain knowledge about various cultures and faiths as they provide support. Asian culture is centered on the extended family, with the entire family making all decisions regarding the patient. Asian-Americans include a diverse group of cultures including, Japanese, Korean, Vietnamese, Chinese, and more. Crying is a form of expression that communicates to others that the griever is feeling the pain of loss. Chinese mourners wail as a sign of suitable mourning (Dowd, Poole, Davidhizar, & Giger. 1998).

A Muslim mourner acknowledges Allah as his or her God. A Muslim may say, "It is the will of Allah" to the deceased person's family. Mourners may wail and scream to express their grief. Cremation is common among Muslims.

Hindus believe that when a person dies, a rebirth takes place. It is believed that the physical body must be cremated in order for the soul to carry on into another incarnation on its karmic journey. Prior to the cremation, the body is washed. Wearing a shroud, the body is surrounded by flowers and carried to the funeral pyre.

Within the Jewish culture, the bodies of deceased Jewish individuals are ritually cleansed by a Jewish individual. The deceased is then dressed in a white linen shroud and placed in a simple wooden casket, which is closed. There is no viewing of the body. The spouse takes full responsibility for making the funeral arrangements, which usually takes place the next day. Years ago, the rabbi would tear a small piece of the mourner's clothing, usually their shirt, to symbolize their mourning. Today, most Jewish mourners wear a torn black ribbon to symbolize being inwardly torn by their grief. The service takes place at the funeral home or at the cemetery and is officiated by a rabbi. The casket will have no flowers covering it.

At the cemetery, Jewish mourners will say the Kaddish prayer that praises God. No stone is placed at the gravesite until 6 months to a year later. This ritual of placing the headstone on the grave is called an unveiling. After the funeral, friends and family return to the mourner's home, which signifies the beginning of the shiva period, which lasts for 7 days. It is customary for anyone who attended the funeral to ritually wash their hands before entering the home. Food is brought from neighbors. Hard-boiled eggs, in particular, symbolize the continuation of life. As signs of mourning, family members sit on low wooden stools and all the mirrors in the home are covered.

Catholics who are dying are given last rites, a ritual of anointing. After death, the body is embalmed and placed in a casket, which may be plain or ornate. For approximately 2 days after the death, mourners, friends and family pay their respects at a vigil. This sharing of time at the funeral home is called a wake, and the casket may be open or closed. Flowers are sent to the funeral home, and Mass cards are left indicating that prayers are being said for the deceased. The funeral is incorporated into the Mass, officiated by a priest, which consists of prayers, bible readings and celebration of the Eucharist. The casket, covered in flowers, is brought to the cemetery in a hearse with the procession of mourners following behind. After the funeral and burial, the family usually goes out to eat together or goes home.

Buddhists look at death and dying in a unique way. Death is considered an awakening, and dying is looked at as being reborn. The dying person's state of mind is of great importance. Friends, family, and monks who recite Buddhist scriptures and mantras usually surround dying Buddhists. This death-related ritual helps the dying person achieve a peaceful state of mind. After a death, Buddhists say prayers, meditate, and do a good deed such as donating to a charity. They can also donate some of the deceased's money to a worthy cause, which allows the deceased to have a good rebirth and attain enlightenment.

> ### Personal Insight
> *What death-related rituals in your culture bring you comfort?*

## Gender Differences

Men and women often grieve in different ways. Stillion and Noviello (2001) noted several differences.

> Therapists, regardless of gender, believed that men and women express grief differently, men and women differ in the coping mechanisms they use for dealing with grief, and friends and acquaintances respond to grieving men and women differently. Specifically, therapists described men's experience of grief as being briefer and their behavior as more stoic, more task oriented, more pragmatic, and less supported than women's experiences (p. 254).

Grieving men may have the public image of strength and control and may want to shield their wives and children. A grieving man may not want to

seek help as he has been conditioned to perceive this as not masculine. Men need to be able to ask for and receive support, and nurses can give them permission to do so. A man and a woman will grieve in their own way; this is especially true after the sudden death of their child. In a study of parents whose children died by accident, homicide, or suicide between the ages of 12 and 28, fathers reported their coping strategies included being restrained and cautious. Mothers reported seeking emotional and instrumental support and turning to religion. This suggests that fathers may be more resigned to the death as it cannot be changed and mothers may be more likely to search for answers and have difficulty accepting the death (Murphy, Johnson, & Weber, 2002).

Widows attempt to find meaning in the loss of their spouses by looking at themselves as survivors with new attitudes and life choices. If bereaved men do not express their grief, they are likely to become marginalized grievers, and the pain of their loss will not be responded to or validated (Zinner, 2000). As men learn to adjust to a world in which their wife is missing, they may experience a decline in health and depression. Whether men accept grief support or not, nurses should continue to offer support and understanding to male grievers.

Although social support diminishes the effects of bereavement, society assumes that men grieve silently and alone (Mastrogianis and Lumley, 2002), The results of their study indicate that bereaved men prefer alternative types of aftercare services such as golf or bowling, cooking classes, legal assistance, and health promotion classes. They found that those men who had a more negative mood were interested in stress management classes. The assumption that men grieve silently and alone may not be true. Nurses help individuals by making recommendations to best fit their style of grieving.

One study examined fathers' grief after the death of a disabled child (Wood and Milo, 2000). The researchers found that grieving fathers wanted to stay busy after the death. Whether these fathers found comfort from sawing down a fallen tree on the day of their child's funeral, choosing the funeral music, or donating their child's retinas and corneas, the father's spoke of "giving their child's life meaning." For these fathers, meaning is found in an action-oriented approach to healing.

After the death of a baby, each parent will grieve in his or her own way. In a bereavement support group, fathers reported that they cried alone in their cars. Wives were not aware that their spouses were crying over the loss of their child. By attending a bereavement support group, spouses were better able to communicate the ways in which they were expressing their grief (Reilly-Smorawski, Armstrong, & Catlin, 2002).

In Rich's study on postpregnancy loss and grief outcome, she found that both husbands and wives equally talked with their family. Though fathers did seek out social support after the loss, more mothers than fathers spoke with their friends and talked with their physician about the reasons for the loss and how to plan for a future pregnancy. Though more mothers than fathers received counseling following the loss, it was the least reported of all services obtained (Rich, 2000).

### Intuitive and Instrumental Grieving Patterns

Conventional-style grievers express their emotions. Society acknowledges the loss by attempting to offer support. Instrumental grievers, whether male or female, do not express their emotions overtly and are less supported by those around them. Instrumental grievers are more cognitive in nature. Any emotional expression would be done in private. Since they do not express their emotions openly, society does not offer them assistance. Being who they are, instrumental grievers would likely reject comfort anyway. Martin and Doka (2000) presented two patterns of grief expression—intuitive and instrumental.

### Intuitive Pattern

1. Feelings are intensely experienced.
2. Expressions such as crying and lamenting mir-

ror inner experience.

3. Successful adaptive strategies facilitate the experience and expression of feelings.
4. There are prolonged periods of confusion, inability to concentrate, disorganization, and disorientation.
5. Physical exhaustion and/or anxiety may result.

### Instrumental Pattern

1. Thinking is predominant to feeling as an experience; feelings are less intense.
2. There is general reluctance to talk about feelings.
3. Mastery of oneself and the environment are most important.
4. Problem solving as a strategy enables mastery of feelings and control of the environment.
5. Brief periods of cognitive dysfunction are common.
6. Energy levels are enhanced, but symptoms of general arousal go unnoticed
(p. 53).

> ### *Personal Insight*
> *Do you consider yourself a conventional, intuitive griever or an instrumental griever?*

### Disenfranchised Grief

The previous section has presented ways grieving individuals feel supported by their spouse, family, clergy, and aftercare services. When an individual experiences a loss, social support is often received from their community. However, there are some losses that are not openly acknowledged, socially supported, or publicly mourned. Doka (1989) defines disenfranchised grief as "the grief that persons experience when they incur a loss that is not or cannot be openly acknowledged, publicly mourned, or socially supported" (p. 4). Society does not look at the loss as significant to that individual, and therefore they cannot actively grieve.

Nurses and other health professionals can be disenfranchised grievers, since people in society and specifically those in their work environment do not recognize the patient's death as a loss to the staff. After a patient dies, caregivers may feel that it is unprofessional for them to reveal their true emotions and that it is not appropriate to grieve their loss (Kaplan, 2000).

---

*Personal Insight*

*If you have ever cried after a patient died, how did your co-workers respond to you as you grieved the patient's death? If you have not experienced the death of a patient, how do you think your coworkers would respond to you if you cried?*

---

A married man having an extramarital affair experiences loss when his lover dies. He grieves her loss but experiences disenfranchised grief, as he cannot share his secret with others. Most likely, no one knew the relationship existed, and he is unable to publicly share the loss. When the death is not socially sanctioned, the individual experiences disenfranchised grief.

When a person dies of AIDS, the bereaved may become disenfranchised grievers as individuals disconnect behaviorally and emotionally from them. The loss of their support system is another loss felt by those who have had loved ones die of AIDS (Ingram, Jones, and Smith, 2001). As of December 2002, 501,669 known AIDS deaths have been reported in the United States. This total includes 496,354 adults and adolescents, 5,315 children under age 15 (National Center for HIV, STD and TB Prevention, 2003). Therefore, this type of disenfranchised grief has likely been experienced by many persons in the United States.

Miscarriages, abortions, and early infant deaths are sometimes missing from the family tree. Though these types of losses occurred, they were probably not openly acknowledged and mourned. After an abortion, a woman may still grieve the loss of her fetus and the loss of her innocence. Though painful, the grief may be disenfranchised, as society did not acknowledge the loss (Gajdos, 2002). Realizing the importance of addressing the loss at

the time it occurs, nurses can help address unresolved feelings. Not much is known about the effect over time of the common life experience of miscarriage or abortion on adolescent women (Wheeler & Austin, 2000). A bereaved adolescent mother may experience disenfranchised grief when she does not get the support needed from her peers. Here again, nurses can play a vital role in providing support to those who grieve.

Children and adolescents are often unrecognized grievers. If a friend or peer dies, their loss is rarely openly acknowledged as adults attempt to shield them from the pain of loss. Another unrecognized griever is the employee who is not given time off to attend a funeral of a close friend. A mentally incompetent individual who is not allowed to attend a service or funeral of a significant person in their life will also face unrecognized grief. Another death that is not socially sanctioned is suicide or autoerotica asphyxia. People may be uncomfortable expressing grief to the mourners due to the type of death, which causes disenfranchised grief. Others who experience disenfranchised grief are ex-spouses, nursing home residents, and suicide survivors. There are special problems for ex-spouses who become disenfranchised in coping with their ex-spouse's terminal illness and dying. When the patient's personal history is taken, it is a good idea to discuss the patient's ex-spouse to fully assess the patient's total needs and address any unresolved issues (Scott, 2000). Those who reside in nursing homes are often grievers who are unrecognized. This is especially true if the resident is terminally ill, their loved one dies, and no one informs them of the death, as shown in the following example.

**Example**

Lois, a terminally ill 62-year-old patient, resides in a facility. Her husband, Nathan, age 64, visits her twice a week. On the morning of his scheduled visit, Nathan suffered a massive heart attack and died. Their son thought it best not to inform Lois of the death and informed the nurse, "Don't tell my mom. It will be too much for her since she is so sick herself." The patient, unaware of the death and not able to attend the funeral, becomes disenfranchised. The nurse explains to the son the importance of being honest with Lois. She attempts to make him understand that Lois, being alert and oriented, will become concerned as to why her husband is not visiting. The lies could cause the patient undue stress, then when and if she finds out, she may experience disenfranchised grief. The nurse said, "Let's be honest with your mom and give her the opportunity to say goodbye. Though she will experience grief, the pain comes from years of loving your dad. We will help her incorporate the loss into the short life that she has left. We will be here to help her cope."

Patients should learn about the death in their family in order to begin grieving (Ufema, 2002).

## Complicated Grief

Grief can become complicated due to several factors. First, the griever's personality has a direct influence on mourning. Grievers who were dependent on the deceased, who were ambivalent toward the deceased, who lacks self-esteem or trust in others, or who have a previous history of psychological vulnerability will experience complications in mourning. If there is a lack of social support and the bereaved feels unsupported, grief can become complicated. Bereavement is a criterion for complicated grief disorder. If an individual experiences a death of a spouse, other relative, or intimate partner and it has been at least 14 months since the death, the grief can be complicated (see Table 2-1).

Sanders (1997) notes certain seriously debilitating risk factors.

- Sudden unexpected deaths, including suicide, murder, catastrophic circumstances, and dependency.
- Parental bereavement.
- Health before bereavement.
- Concurrent crisis.
- Perceived lack of social support.

- Age and gender.
- Reduced material resources.

Prigerson et al. (2002) point out that complicated grief symptoms were found in those whose family members died in a violent way. Their symptoms were longing, yearning, anger, and bitterness. Complicated grief symptoms were also found in those whose family members died from a health problem or surgery. The bereaved felt pain in the same part of body as their loved one. Other symptoms included being envious of those who were not

### TABLE 2-1: PROPOSED CRITERIA FOR COMPLICATED GRIEF DISORDER

**Event Criterion/Prolonged Response Criterion**

Bereavement (loss of a spouse, other relative, or intimate partner)

At least 14 months ago (12 months is avoided because of possible intense turbulence from an anniversary reaction)

**Signs and Symptoms Criteria**

In the last month, any three of the following seven symptoms with a severity that interferes with daily functioning

*Intrusive symptoms*

1. Unbidden memories or intrusive fantasies related to the lost relationship
2. Strong spells or pangs of severe emotion related to the lost relationship
3. Distressingly strong yearnings or wishes that the deceased were there

*Signs of avoidance and failure to adapt*

4. Feelings of being far too much alone or personally empty
5. Excessively staying away from people, places, or activities that remind the subject of the deceased
6. Unusual levels of sleep disturbances
7. Loss of interest in work, social, caretaking, or recreational activities to a maladaptive degree

*Source:* Horowitz, Siegel, Holen, Bonanno, Milbrath, & Stinson (1997), Diagnostic criteria for complicated grief disorder, *Am J Psychiatry, 154,* 904-910.

bereaved. They could not imagine being fulfilled and felt a loss sense of security and trust.

Rando (1984) notes the various forms of unresolved grief. She maintains that forms of complicated grief include absent grief, defined as inhibition of typical expression of grief. Delayed grief is defined as a significant period of time (e.g., weeks to years) between the loss and the onset of grief reaction. Prolonged, chronic, or unresolved grief includes a prolonged persistent depression and preoccupation with the loss, with intense yearnings for the deceased that continue over time.

Rando (1993) maintains that the six "R" processes of mourning needed for healthy accommodation of loss are:

- recognizing the loss,

- reacting to the separation,

- recollecting and reexperiencing the deceased and the relationship,

- relinquishing the old attachments to the deceased and the old assumptive world,

- readjusting to move adaptively into the new world without forgetting the old, and

- reinvesting.

Complicated mourning takes place when there is a compromise, distortion, or failure of one or more of the six "R" processes of mourning. In the recognition process, the grieving individual acknowledges and understands that the death took place and experiences the pain of that loss. In reacting, they feel the loss and express it and also mourn the secondary losses associated with the death of their loved one. They then review and remember times shared with their loved one and re-experience the feelings associated with those thoughts. To relinquish their hold, they revise their assumptive world, develop a new relationship with their loved one, adapt new ways of being in their world, and form a new identity. Rando maintains:

The process is lengthy because only by bumping up against the new world and discovering that the old assumptions, expectations, and beliefs–and the needs, feelings, thoughts, behavior and interaction patterns, hopes, wishes, fantasies, and dreams that coincide with them–no longer fit does the mourner learn the lesson that they must be changed (p. 428).

If, after the death of a significant person, some responses are marked and persistent for at least 2 months that cause significant impairment in functioning, the individual may be experiencing traumatic grief (see Table 2-2), which is defined as a "disorder that occurs after the death of a significant other. Symptoms of separation distress are the core of the disorder and amalgamate with bereavement specific symptoms of being devastated and traumatized by the death" (Jacobs, 1999, p. 24). The death does not necessarily occur under a traumatic circumstance. Risk factors include losses that are sudden, unexpected, or disenfranchised. Various risk factors include kinship (e.g., death of parents) the nature of the loss, being unprepared, multiple losses, violent death, and feelings of responsibility, whether personal or displaced on others.

To meet the needs of individuals grieving, health professionals can review how they have reacted to the loss and the factors that influence their reactions. Some of the factors include the circumstances of the event, the nature of the relationship, the interaction between survivor and society, and the physical condition of the body. Prigerson et al. (1997) suggested mental health professionals intervene at 6 months after the death. Horowitz et al. (1997) found that intervention should take place after 12 months. A recent study (Ott & Lueger, 2002) found that professionals should assess the bereaved for complicated bereavement not only at 6 months, but also at 9, 12, 15, and 18 months or later.

## TABLE 2-2: PROPOSED CRITERIA FOR TRAUMATIC GRIEF

### Criterion A

1. The person has experienced the death of a significant other.

2. The response involves intrusive, distressing preoccupation with the deceased person (e.g. yearning, longing, or searching).

### Criterion B

In response to the death, the following symptom(s) is/are marked and persistent:

1. Frequent efforts to avoid reminders of the deceased (e.g., thoughts, feelings, activities, people, places)

2. Purposelessness or feelings of futility about the future

3. Subjective sense of numbness, detachment, or absence of emotional responsiveness

4. Feeling stunned, dazed, or shocked

5. Difficulty acknowledging the death (e.g., disbelief)

6. Feeling that life is empty or meaningless

7. Difficulty imagining a fulfilling life without the deceased

8. Feeling that part of oneself has died

9. Shattered worldview (e.g., lost sense of security, trust, or control)

10. Assumes symptoms or harmful behaviors of, or related to, the deceased person

11. Excessive irritability, bitterness, or anger related to the death

### Criterion C

The duration of the disturbance (symptoms listed) is at least two months.

### Criterion D

The disturbance causes clinically significant impairment in social, occupational, or other important areas of functioning.

*Source:* Jacobs, S., Mazure, C., & Prigerson, H. (2000). Diagnostic criteria for traumatic grief. *Death Studies,* 24(3), p. 189.

## Bereavement

Where grief is the personalized feelings and emotional response to loss, bereavement is the time of being deprived of that which we have valued. We value a person's life and there is a state of sorrow due to the death of that person. Usually there is a time period associated with the death called the bereavement period. It is during this time the survivors, otherwise known as the bereaved, mourn the loss and grieve.

## Mourning

Rando (2000) and Corr, Nabe, and Corr (2000) suggest that grief is the reactive response to loss, while mourning encompasses a series of actions undertaken to accommodate the loss within a person's life. Stroebe, Stroebe, and Hanson (1997) define mourning as "the actions and manner of expressing grief, which often reflect the mourning practices of one's culture" (p. 5).

The role of the nurse in providing support to those who mourn will depend upon the situation. Although nurses are not bereavement counselors, virtually every nurse deals with some issues of death, dying, grief, bereavement, and mourning. Nurses will be more effective in providing support if they understand mourning. Mourning is the expression that refers to the period of time when grief goes public, when people may wear black clothes or a black arm band. In the outward expression of loss, those who mourn adjust to the realities of what has happened.

Nurses can make those who mourn aware that mourning is a process that takes time. Though there will be some good days, there will also be bad ones. Rando (1993) reported that the initial process of mourning includes recognizing that the loss has occurred. After the grieving individual understands that their loved one is really dead, mourning the loss begins. Though being active and forming new relationships eases the pain, the person who died can never be substituted.

Grieving individuals behave in a certain way, and their customs vary depending upon their culture. This cultural influence can play a part the decision of the bereaved to begin dating. It also plays a role in their choice of clothing, whether to wear black and at what point to return to wearing clothing worn prior to the death. No matter what the mourning custom, ceremony, or ritual, nurses must always show respect to their patients and family members. Death-related ceremonies and rituals bring comfort to those who mourn. After the death of a patient, nurses can be most helpful when discussing death-related ceremonies and rituals with their patient's family members. A nurse can say, "I am very sorry for your loss. It is a difficult time. Perhaps in your culture there are certain mourning rituals. May I ask, what are some of your mourning rituals?" Those who mourn can then reflect on ways to cope with the pain of loss.

## Four Tasks of Mourning

According to Worden (2002), abnormal grief reactions occur when people are unable to complete the four tasks of mourning. First, the grieving person must accept the reality of the loss. In accepting the reality, the bereaved understands their loved one is truly dead. If the death is unexpected, they may experience denial and find it difficult to accept that the person is really dead and will not return. For actualization of the death to take place, the mourner can:

- view the body before the funeral,
- attend the service and/or funeral,
- visit the cemetery,
- view photographs and personal belongings of the deceased,
- give some of the clothes, jewelry, and belongings of the deceased to friends and relatives.

The second task of mourning is working through the pain of grief. The bereaved may attempt to numb the pain with illegal drugs and alcohol. They may work long hours to avoid the deep pain of loss. They experience physical and emotional pain. For some, the pain is so great that they attempt to avoid it by not visiting places their loved one may have been. However, after the death of a loved one, it is impossible to not to feel the pain of that loss. Sooner or later, the pain will be felt and grief experienced.

The third task of mourning is adjusting to an environment in which the deceased is missing. If the individual does not adjust, he or she may withdraw from life. Bereaved individuals have new responsibilities and must take on roles their loved one used to perform. The spouse realizes that the loved one is dead every time they do a chore their loved one used to do, even simply taking out the garbage. If the grieving wife has never driven a car, she may need to take lessons and learn how to drive. If her husband prepared the yearly taxes, she must learn how to do the taxes or find ways to get them done. The widowed, therefore, take on new responsibilities and must not withdraw from life.

The fourth and final task of mourning is when the individual emotionally relocates the deceased and moves on with life. The bereaved develops healthy new relationships with others. However, by doing so, he or she may feel disloyal to the deceased loved one. Their task is to create new relationships while not forgetting their loved one. Widowers may seek out another wife. A woman may decide to get pregnant after the death of her baby. It may be difficult to emotionally relocate the deceased.

Although the bereaved person may need to invest in new relationships, he or she may not be able to do so. Establishing new relationships causes the person to be vulnerable. This new relationship may end. It opens him or her up to the possibility that this new relationship may end or that the person may die and fear another experience of loss. Once the final task of mourning is complete, the grieving person emotionally relocates the deceased and moves on with his or her life.

Neimeyer (2000) expanded the tasks of mourning as a set of challenges to the mourner to

1. acknowledge the reality of the loss,

2. open yourself to the pain,

3. revise your assumptive world,

4. reconstruct your relationship to that which has been lost,

5. reinvent yourself.

## Meaning Making

*The mystery of life, cloaked so guilelessly in day and night, makes the search for God the enduring human drama. We know so little, we feel so much. We have only the shape of our lives, experienced in the cycle of light and dark, to guide us toward meaning.*

— Hampl, 1995, p. xxvi

When a loved one or significant other dies, those grieving the loss will react to that loss and attempt to find meaning in it. Making meaning is defined "generally as finding some degree of coherence, orderliness, predictability, purpose or value in what happened" (Gamino, Hogan, & Sewell, 2002, p. 794). Meaning protects us from the fear of dying and what comes after our death. Murphy, Clark-Johnson, and Lohan (2003) found that one of the predictors of parents finding meaning 5 years after the death of a child was the use of religious coping. Meaning is made as the person establishes an understanding of the situation (O'Connor, 2002-2003).

Strategies are needed to understand that a loved one is no longer alive and physically present. The grieving individual attempts to understand the circumstances around the death and the situation. The person tries to cope with the fact that the person is really dead. The bereaved had a bond and shared a relationship. Though the person is dead, a healthy connection can still be maintained. Attig (1996) notes that the bereaved can relearn their relationship with the deceased. The love felt does not die, and the relationship is not dead. The bereaved can continue to hold close those who die even though the person is no longer alive. The author maintains that

letting go entirely is not necessary. The bereaved should not fear being morbid if they continue to talk about their loved one or decide to keep the clothes of the deceased. This experience can even be life-affirming, as meaning is found in the sharing of stories and the act of smelling of or touching the clothes worn by the deceased.

Meaning is also found as the bereaved carries on in the absence of the deceased. Life is for them not over even though the person they cared for is dead. Life goes on, and decisions still must be made. However, these choices and decisions can be made with the deceased in mind. Promises made to the deceased are kept and by so doing, the bereaved continue to maintain the connection. Attig (1996) tells us that as stories of the deceased are shared, the bereaved individual becomes self-transformed and inspired. There is a spiritual connection and a reason and purpose in life as well as death. The bereaved attempts to create some type of order in life to keep their world cohesive and predictable. A nurse can support the bereaved by acknowledging the purpose of their life and the purpose in continuing the relationship with the deceased.

The different grief theories enumerated in this chapter explain how grieving individuals can be supported. Despite the disparity between the theories mentioned, there appears to be one element that is common to all, the maintaining of the relationship with the deceased. The bond between the deceased and the living is permanent and eternal. It is normal for survivors to maintain an inner representation of the deceased and to hold the deceased in loving memory forever (Klass, Silverman, & Nickman, 1996). The continued confidence that the bond they shared will never be broken brings comfort and support to those who grieve.

The essential purpose of continuing the spiritual bonds is to enable the griever to develop a new and meaningful relationship with the deceased. Parkes (2003) notes that in regard to continuing the bonds,

My own view is that there is a literal truth in the statement, "He or she lives on in my memory," but it is important for bereaved people to discover which habits of thought and behavior are now obsolete and must be let go and which can be retained (p. 39).

Thoughts and behaviors that bring comfort change as time passes. However, the connection remains. Survivors sense their loved one's presence through memories and feelings, and this continues the spiritual connection with the deceased (Gamino et al., 2002). Grieving individuals have reported that they felt the deceased was "watching over them" and there was still an "inner connection" to their loved one (Gamino, 2002). This inner connection is particularly felt when grieving individuals create death rituals.

## Death-Related Ceremonies and Rituals

Death rituals are a response to a loss situation and bring comfort to those who mourn. Rituals may be defined as ceremonial actions that have meaning and significance to the individual performing, or observing the act. One death-related ceremony is a eulogy. As mourners gather together, eulogies are said. In these final moments, respect is paid as words are spoken about the deceased, the relationships shared, and the meaning of their life.

Ceremonies and rituals provide support to those who are dying and to those who are present during their last moments. Health professionals must be aware of the importance of these death-related healing experiences. By appreciating their significance, professionals are better able to understand what is significant to the patient and to the family members. These rituals offer the bereaved a last opportunity to prepare the body and visit with the deceased. Depending upon the religion of the deceased, rituals can include:

1. anointing the body with oil,

2. writing obituaries to share the loss with the community, and

3. sitting vigil, where the loved ones recognize the patient is dying or has died. Music can be played, candles lit, and prayers said, as those who cared for the patient say their last goodbyes.

Richards, Wrubel, & Folkman (1999-2000) note three times of death rituals:

1. grooming and preparing the body,

2. ceremonies of transition and separation, and

3. visitations with the deceased (p. 340).

If grieving individuals do not have any rituals, they can invent them (Sanders, 2001). Through our inventions we create something meaningful that sustains us as we reflect upon the loss in our lives. Pollack (2003) pointed out that "in the aftermath of tragedy, memorials and gravesites are frequently constructed. From the tombs of the unknown warrior to the cemeteries in Normandy, memorials and rituals are commonly constructed in the aftermath of tragedy" (p. 125).

> ### *Personal Insight*
> *Is there a patient in particular whose death you grieved? Did you create any type of ritual to recognize their death?*

After 9/11, mourners created rituals that represented their grief. These rituals empowered those who were grieving. Doka (2003) maintains:

Rituals permit meaningful action at a disorganized time; it allows people to "do something." By doing something, even engaging in ritual, we feel that we have symbolic mastery over events. Ritual allows a reorganization of community and continuity in a chaotic time. Collectively, it offers a reassurance that while we cannot control the tragedy itself, we have reasserted control in its aftermath (p. 180).

Doka (2003) describes spontaneous rituals, planned rituals, ongoing rituals, and therapeutic rituals as four kinds of rituals in public tragedy. After the September 11th public tragedy, many

Americans donated to those intimately affected by the terrorist attack. The tragic deaths of thousands of men and women brought about many spontaneous rituals. Survivors felt a need to do something positive, which helped them cope with the situation.

A planned ritual can be a private ritual, which honors a person who died, an organizational ritual, which honors a victim of that organization, or a public ritual, which brings grieving communities together. One ongoing ritual usually takes place on the anniversary of the event. When sharing ongoing rituals during the anniversary period, individuals come together and reflect on the event, those who lost their lives, and those who mourn them. Examples of a therapeutic ritual include writing a letter, planting a tree, or lighting a candle.

Like rituals, spontaneous memorials are immediate expressions of grief. Permanent memorials are lasting impressions and acknowledgements at the site. Roadside death memorials (RDMs) bring comfort to the bereaved. After a motor vehicle accident, they may leave crosses, flowers, ribbons, notes, or other mementos at the site of the accident. These artifacts are reminders to all who pass the site that someone special died due to a collision there. As a memorialization, RDMs provide a way to express intense grief and are a means of communication with and about the deceased (Reid & Reid, 2001)

### Role of Symbolic Representation

When individuals are in mourning, they are comforted by reminders of their loved ones. Certain objects that the bereaved once owned become very significant. Schuchter and Zisook (1988), define symbolic representation as "a process wherein possessions, creations, or shared experiences of the deceased are imbued with the spirit or memories of the dead, a process that evolves before the death but develops a higher valence only after the death." The symbolic representations connect us to the dead and become a linking object (Vickio, 1999—see Figure 2-1).

## FIGURE 2-1: THE ROLE OF SYMBOLIC REPRESENTATIONS

Objects that have the power to link us to the deceased can include items such as videotapes and photographs that graphically capture the image of the deceased. Personal items that were either created or routinely used by the deceased can also serve to remind us of our loved ones and allow us to feel close to them. Sometimes these connecting objects can take a less concrete form—for instance, we might find that a particular aroma or melody links us powerfully to the memory of the deceased.

In my personal life, I have a number of cherished possessions that connect me to deceased loved ones. One such item is a psychological testing instrument, the Thematic Apperception Test (Murray, 1943). This instrument was given to me by the widow of one of my graduate school mentors following his death. (The deceased professor had been my instructor for two classes, my clinical supervisor, a member of my research committee, and an occasional tennis partner.) When I now use the test in assessing clients, I find myself looking at my mentor's handwritten instructions on the outside of the test box; I can imagine him reading these instructions aloud and can vividly envision him administering the test. At such times, I am strongly reminded of how much I continue to feel my mentor's presence in my life and my work.

*Source:* Vickio, C.J. (1999). Together in spirit: Keeping our relationships alive when loved ones die. *Death Studies, 23*:161-175.

# SUMMARY

This chapter examined the factors that influence the grief process. The chapter highlighted grief's origins and defined it as a process that includes the intense physical, emotional, and spiritual suffering after a loss. The physical, emotional, cognitive, psychological, behavioral, religious, and cultural factors that influence grief were explored. Ways that Asians, Muslims, Hindus, Buddhists, Catholics, and Jews deal with death were examined.

The next part of this chapter examined some of the gender differences after a child dies. One study examined a father's grief after his disabled child dies and how meaning is found in an action-oriented approach to healing. Ways that intuitive and instrumental grievers express their grief were explored. Post-pregnancy loss and grief outcome were highlighted. How parents cope in their own way after the sudden death of a child by accident, homicide, or suicide was explored along with how widows attempt to find meaning in the loss of their spouses.

Disenfranchised grief was defined and examples offered to show the challenges for those who have incurred a loss that cannot be openly acknowledged, publicly mourned, or socially supported. Nurses can be disenfranchised grievers, as society does not recognize the patient's death as a loss to the staff. Some of the examples of disenfranchised grief included a married man having an extramarital affair who experiences the death of his lover; a person who dies of AIDS in the face of a social stigma and individuals who disconnect behaviorally and emotionally from the survivors; women who suffer miscarriages, abortions, and early infant deaths; children and adolescents who may be prevented from grieving in an attempt to protect them; and survivors of those who died by suicide or autoerotica asphyxia.

This chapter identified bereavement and mourning, and the risk factors for complicated grief were highlighted. Rando's six "R" processes of mourning, needed for healthy accommodation of loss, were noted. Current theories of grief and mourning were identified. Worden's four tasks of mourning—whereby the grieving person must accept the reality of the loss, work through the pain of grief, adjust to an environment in which the deceased is missing, and emotionally relocate the deceased and move on with life—were discussed. It was noted how Neimeyer expanded the tasks as a set of challenges to the mourner. Attig's strategies that are helpful in maintaining a healthy connection to the deceased were examined. By stressing several different theo-

ries, it was explained how grieving individuals can be supported. The essential purpose of continuing the spiritual bonds to enable the griever to develop a new and meaningful relationship with the deceased was noted.

The chapter discussed the definition of mourning and how customs vary depending upon the grieving individual's culture. The significance of death-related ceremonies and rituals and the importance of death-related healing experiences were noted. A description of spontaneous rituals, planned rituals, public rituals, ongoing rituals, and therapeutic rituals after a public tragedy was given. Spontaneous memorials were explained as immediate expressions of grief. Finally, the role of symbolic representation—wherein possessions, creations, or shared experiences of the deceased develops a higher value after the death—was noted.

# RESOURCES

## The Grief Process on the Internet

AARP: Grief and Loss
   www.aarp.org/griefandloss

The Association for Death Education and
   Counseling (ADEC)
   www.adec.org

Grief Share: Finding help as you grieve the loss.
   www.griefshare.org

Grief Net: Grief Process on the Internet: An
   Internet community of persons dealing with
   grief, death, and major loss.
   http://griefnet.org

Grief Recovery: The action program for moving
   beyond loss — Certification Training.
   www.grief-recovery.com

# EXAM QUESTIONS

## CHAPTER 2
**Questions 11-24**

11. The process that includes the intense physical, emotional, and spiritual suffering after a loss is called

    a. grief.
    b. bereavement.
    c. mourning.
    d. death.

12. The pattern of expression of an intuitive griever is

    a. thinking is predominant to feeling as an experience.
    b. feelings are less intense.
    c. a general reluctance to talk about feelings.
    d. feelings are intensely and overtly experienced.

13. Individuals who express their grief through an instrumental pattern

    a. have a greater reluctance to talk about their feelings.
    b. express themselves through crying.
    c. are physically exhausted.
    d. do not experience their feelings intensely.

14. The type of grief persons experience when they incur a loss that is not or cannot be openly acknowledged, publicly mourned, or socially supported is

    a. marginalized.
    b. disenfranchised.
    c. complicated.
    d. traumatic.

15. An intrusive symptom of complicated grief disorder is

    a. distressingly strong yearnings or wishes that the deceased were there.
    b. feeling that life is empty or meaningless.
    c. excessive irritability, bitterness, or anger related to the death.
    d. feeling that part of oneself has died.

16. A seriously debilitating risk factor in grief is

    a. cultural issues.
    b. concurrent crisis.
    c. health after bereavement.
    d. increased material resources.

17. Grief that involves a significant period of time from the loss to the onset of a grief reaction is

    a. complicated grief.
    b. delayed grief.
    c. exaggerated grief.
    d. disenfranchised grief.

18. The time in which we experience a state of sorrow as we feel deprived of a person we have valued is

    a. grief.

    b. mourning.

    c. bereavement.

    d. culture.

19. Shared social expressions or acts that show one's grief in a given society or cultural group is

    a. bereavement.

    b. mourning.

    c. death.

    d. culture.

20. According to Rando, during the initial process of mourning the survivors

    a. revive their assumptive world.

    b. recognize that the loss has occurred.

    c. accept the reality of the loss.

    d. suffer disenfranchised grief.

21. According to Worden, the bereaved who are unable to complete the four tasks of mourning experience

    a. abnormal grief reactions.

    b. crying.

    c. sighing.

    d. adjusting to an environment in which the loved one is missing.

22. For actualization of the death to take place, the mourner

    a. numbs the pain with illegal drugs and alcohol.

    b. denies the death took place.

    c. views photographs and personal belongings of the deceased.

    d. gives up customs and traditions.

23. An individual who attempts to numb the pain with illegal drugs and alcohol or by working long hours to avoid the deep pain of loss is trying to avoid the task of

    a. accepting the reality of the loss.

    b. working through the pain of grief.

    c. adjusting to an environment in which the deceased is missing.

    d. emotionally relocating the deceased and moving on with life.

24. Individuals who take on roles their loved one used to perform are involved in the mourning task of

    a. accepting the reality of the loss.

    b. working through the pain of grief.

    c. adjusting to an environment in which the deceased is missing.

    d. emotionally relocating the deceased and moving on with life.

# CHAPTER 3

# SUICIDE AND LIFE-THREATENING BEHAVIOR

## CHAPTER OBJECTIVE

After completing this chapter, the reader will be able to identify the types of suicide, risk factors for suicide, and the differences between suicide prevention, intervention, and postvention.

## LEARNING OBJECTIVES:

After studying this chapter, the reader will be able to

1. recognize risk factors and warning signs for suicide.

2. differentiate between suicide prevention and suicide intervention.

3. distinguish between physician-assisted suicide and euthanasia.

4. choose ways to support survivors of suicide.

## SUICIDE

Figures from the National Center for Health Statistics (Anderson, 2002) estimate that 29,350 Americans complete suicide each year. The suicide process begins with suicide ideation. The person ruminates about the idea of suicide, possibly makes a verbal or written threat of suicide, and may end with the completed act. Gutierrez, Rodriguez, and Garcia (2001) define *suicide* as

a death by self-inflicted means where there is evidence that the intent was to cause death. *Suicide attempts* are nonfatal acts, with or without injury, where there is evidence that the person had some intent to cause death. *Suicide threat* may be spoken or unspoken, does not involve a self-harmful act, but the intention is to communicate that a specific act of self-harm may happen soon (p. 320).

Many who have attempted suicide pass through their local emergency rooms. The emergency room nurse must be confident in evaluating the suicidal patient and making sure a mental health professional and, if possible, a psychiatrist will see the patient.

A suicide assessment should never be postponed to future meetings. It is also critical to have someone stay with the patient. Many hospitals hire sitters to stay with the patient, and these sitters inform the nurse immediately if the patient appears ready to hurt themselves. Such sitters do not require any formal medical training. If no sitter is available, the patient should be visible at all times. Rather than having the psychiatrist see the patient at the end of the medical workup, the patient should be seen periodically throughout their time in the E.R. to see any changes in behavior.

As a health professional cultivates a therapeutic alliance with a suicidal patient, an assessment is made using the risk factors for suicide (see Table 3-1).

## Psychological Explanations of Suicide

Lack of coping skills and problem-solving ability may be factors for increased depression and suicide ideation (Olvera, 2001). The psychological explanations of suicide stem from the individual's needs not being met. If the individual does not cope with the psychological pain caused by the frustration of these needs, they may complete suicide. One other psychological explanation includes having tunnel vision, in that the suicidal person only sees one way of coping with the problem. Hirschfeld and Russell

(1997) list clinical risk factors as hopelessness, clinical depression or schizophrenia, substance abuse, history of suicide ideation, panic attacks, and severe anhedonia. Due to the tunnel vision, the person focuses on the problem and can't cope with it, which can lead to suicide. This is especially true for schizophrenics, who feel helpless, inadequate, and may not tell anyone that they are contemplating suicide (see

### TABLE 3-1: SUICIDE RISK FACTORS

- Previous suicide attempt
- Mental disorders—particularly mood disorders such as depression and bipolar disorder
- Co-occurring mental and alcohol and substance abuse disorders
- Family history of suicide
- Hopelessness
- Impulsive and/or aggressive tendencies
- Barriers to accessing mental health treatment
- Relational, social, work, or financial loss
- Physical illness
- Easy access to lethal methods, especially guns
- Unwillingness to seek help because of stigma attached to mental and substance abuse disorders and/or suicidal thoughts
- Influence of significant people—family members, celebrities, peers who have died by suicide—both through direct personal contact or inappropriate media representations
- Cultural and religious beliefs—for instance, the belief that suicide is a noble resolution of a personal dilemma
- Local epidemics of suicide that have a contagious influence
- Isolation, a feeling of being cut off from other people

*Source:* U.S. Public Health Service. (1999). *The Surgeon General's call to action to prevent suicide.* Washington DC: Dept. of Health & Human Services. Available online: http://www.surgeongeneral.gov/library/call toaction/calltoaction.htm

### FIGURE 3-1: SCHIZOPHRENIA AND SUICIDE

Schizophrenia, the most chronic and disabling of the severe mental disorders, is a major focus of research at the National Institute of Mental Health (NIMH), the world's foremost mental health scientific organization. This Federal agency takes the lead in neuroscientific investigation devoted to understanding the causes, diagnosis, prevention, and treatment of schizophrenia and other mental disorders, which afflict millions of Americans.

Since the Institute's inception 50 years ago, much has been learned about mental disorders and their effects on the brain. Revolutionary scientific advances in neuroscience, molecular biology, genetics, and brain imaging have provided some of the greatest insights into the complex organ that is the seat of thought, memory, and emotion. Thanks to these new tools, the scientific evidence that mental illnesses are brain disorders exists.

More than 2 million Americans are affected by schizophrenia. The illness, which may impair a person's ability to manage emotions, interact with others, and think clearly, typically develops in the late teens or early twenties. Symptoms include hallucinations, delusions, disordered thinking, and social withdrawal. Most people with schizophrenia continue to suffer chronically or episodically throughout their lives. Even between bouts of active illness, lost opportunities for careers and relationships, stigma, residual symptoms, and medication side effects often plague those with the illness. One of every 10 people with schizophrenia eventually commits suicide.

*Source:* Dept. of Health & Human Services, National Institute of Mental Health. (2000). Fact Sheet: Schizophrenia research. NIMH Publication No. 00-4500, May 2000. http://www.nimh.nih.gov/publicat/schizresfact.cfm

Figure 3-1). Donatelle (2003) notes that schizophrenia is characterized by "alterations of the senses (including auditory and visual hallucinations); the inability to sort out incoming stimuli and make appropriate responses; an altered sense of self; and radical changes in emotions, movements, and behaviors" (p. 45). Individuals who are schizophrenic have a high rate of suicide (Fenton, 2000; Roy, 2001).

Those living with cancer may also be at a greater risk for suicide. The stressful situation of living with a life-threatening disease such as cancer may cause symptoms of depression, hopelessness, and suicide ideation (Gilbar & Eden, 2000). Another group with a greater risk for suicide is adults who were maltreated as children. Gibb et al. (2001) examined childhood maltreatment and college students' current suicide ideation and found that the students who were emotionally maltreated in childhood had higher levels of suicide ideation across the 2.5 year follow-up.

The elderly form the group with the greatest risk for suicide. In a study of 83 elderly people in a nursing home, they reported high levels of depression, suicidality, and hopelessness. Loneliness is also an important variable when incidence of suicidal behavior is concerned. These residents attempt to cope with the changes in their social life and family status. Those who reside in nursing homes are just as likely to die by suicide as those who do not live in nursing facilities. Their risk factors include both a sense of loss and disabilities (Ron, 2002).

## Biological Explanations of Suicide

Overall, males are four times more likely to complete suicide than females (Centers for Disease Control & Prevention [CDC]; National Center for Injury Prevention & Control [NCIPC], 2000). Although it is widely accepted that many people who died by suicide have a psychiatric disorder, there can also be biological explanations of suicide. Suicide ideation can be due to diminished function of the brain's neurotransmitter serotonin (Roy,

2001). This biochemical imbalance can lead to suicide ideation (see Table 3-2). Those at elevated risk for suicide are individuals with affective disorders, bipolar disorders, and alcoholism and substance abuse diagnoses.

### TABLE 3-2: THE LINKS BETWEEN DEPRESSION AND SUICIDE

- Major depression is the psychiatric diagnosis most commonly associated with suicide.
- About 2/3 of people who complete suicide are depressed at the time of their deaths.
- One out of every 16 people who are diagnosed with depression eventually go on to end their lives through suicide.
- About 7 out of every 100 men and 1 out of every 100 women who have been diagnosed with depression in their lifetime will go on to complete suicide.
- The risk of suicide in people with major depression is about 20 times that of the general population.
- People who have had multiple episodes of depression are at greater risk for suicide than those who have had one episode.
- People who have a dependence on alcohol or drugs in addition to being depressed are at greater risk for suicide.
- People who are depressed and exhibit the following symptoms are at particular risk for suicide:
  1. Extreme hopelessness
  2. A lack of interest in activities that were previously pleasurable
  3. Heightened anxiety and/or panic attacks
  4. Global insomnia
  5. Talk about suicide or a prior history of attempts/acts
  6. Irritability and agitation

*Source:* American Association of Suicidology. *The links between depression and suicide.* Washington, D.C. Available online: http://www.suicidology.org/displaycommon.cfm?an=1&subarticlenbr=31

## Sociological Explanations of Suicide

The first study of suicide was by Emile Durkheim in 1897. Durkheim (1897, 1951) maintained that the social suicide rate was defined by two distinct social characteristics. The first characteristic is the degree of social integration where individuals are bound together in a society. The second characteristic is the degree of social regulation where the individual's emotions, desires, and behaviors are governed by the norms of society. Suicide rates will be higher when social integration is too high or too low. If social integration is too high it can lead to altruistic suicide, and if too low, it can lead to egotistic suicide. When the level of social regulation is too high, it can lead to fatalistic suicide, and when the level is too low, it can lead to anomic suicide. In a fatalistic suicide, people believe they have no future due to political or economic expression. In anomic suicide, people are in a crisis situation and are confused due to major changes in their society. They are unable to cope with the rules and the changes, such as economic problems. These individuals don't know what is expected of them, believe their life has no value in their society, and they kill themselves.

Lester (1999) described that the primary purpose of *altruistic* suicide is in the name of peace. Altruistic suicide occurs when a person has unselfish motives, being so integrated into a particular social group, that they believe it is their duty to die for that group. Craig Badiali and Joan Fox were two teenagers who completed suicide in 1969 to protest the Vietnam War (Asinof, 1971). These two New Jersey students died, perhaps believing that their death would benefit society by creating peace. Marilyn Monroe's death, however, was an *egotistic* suicide. She was alone, perhaps feeling as though she was not part of any group. Corr et al. (2003) note, "Egotistic suicide depends on an underinvolvement or underintegration, a kind of disintegration and isolation of an individual from his or her society" (p. 470). Examples of *fatalistic* suicide, where the individual believes they have no future,

were that of Sigmund Freud who was dying of cancer, and Ernest Hemingway, who feared being placed in an institution. Freddie Prinze, an addict, and Virginia Woolf, who feared she was going insane, are examples of *anomic* suicides, where the person in a crisis situation does not see any solution to their problems. Corr et al. note other examples of anomic suicide:

> In contemporary American society, examples of this sort of suicide might involve adolescents who have been unexpectedly rejected by a peer group, some farmers who find that economic and social forces outside their control are forcing them into bankruptcy and taking away both their livelihood and their way of life, or middle-aged employees who have developed specialized work skills and who have devoted themselves for years to their employer only to be suddenly thrown out of the jobs and economically dislocated. For such individuals, underregulation or a sudden withdrawal of control may be intolerable because of the absence of (familiar) principles to guide them in living (p. 471).

Several researchers have noted the sociological explanations of suicide. Hirschfeld and Russell (1997) list sociodemographic risk factors as those who are unemployed, white or Native American, widowed, males over the age of 60 who are living alone, and those having financial problems with a recent loss. Orbach, Stein, Shani-Sela, and Har-Even (2001) studied three groups of adolescents from ages 14-18. They reported that there was a relationship between negative attitudes toward their body and suicide ideation. McBee-Strayer & Rogers (2002) studied 162 adult lesbians, gays, and bisexuals: 41% reported seriously considering suicide and had a suicide plan, 36% reported past suicide attempts, and 46% reported they might attempt suicide in the future. What these studies show is that each person needs to have a place in our community and in our society. We need to feel, and be accepted as, a part of that group.

## FIGURE 3-2: A LETTER FROM THE SURGEON GENERAL

### U.S. Department of Health and Human Services

Suicide is a serious public health problem. In 1996, the year for which the most recent statistics are available, suicide was the ninth leading cause of mortality in the United States, responsible for nearly 31,000 deaths. This number is more than 50% higher than the number of homicides in the United States in the same year (around 20,000 homicides in 1996). Many fail to realize that far more Americans die from suicide than from homicide. Each year in the United States, approximately 500,000 people require emergency room treatment as a result of attempted suicide. Suicidal behavior typically occurs in the presence of mental or substance abuse disorders—illnesses that impose their own direct suffering. Suicide is an enormous trauma for millions of Americans who experience the loss of someone close to them. The nation must address suicide as a significant public health problem and put into place national strategies to prevent the loss of life and the suffering suicide causes.

In 1996, the World Health Organization (WHO), recognizing the growing problem of suicide worldwide, urged member nations to address suicide. Its document, *Prevention of Suicide: Guidelines for the Formulation and Implementation of National Strategies*, motivated the creation of an innovative public/private partnership to seek a national strategy for the United States. This public/private partnership included agencies in the U.S. Department of Health and Human Services, encompassing the Centers for Disease Control and Prevention (CDC), the Health Resources and Services Administration (HRSA), the Indian Health Service (IHS), the National Institute of Mental Health (NIMH), the Office of the Surgeon General, and the Substance Abuse and Mental Health Services Administration (SAMHSA) and the Suicide Prevention Advocacy Network (SPAN), a public grassroots advocacy organization made up of suicide survivors (persons close to someone who completed suicide), attempters of suicide, community activists, and health and mental health clinicians.

An outgrowth of this collaborative effort was a jointly sponsored national conference on suicide prevention convened in Reno, Nevada, in October 1998. Conference participants included researchers, health and mental health clinicians, policy makers, suicide survivors, and community activists and leaders. They engaged in careful analysis of what is known and unknown about suicide and its potential responsiveness to a public health model emphasizing suicide prevention.

This *Surgeon General's Call To Action* introduces a blueprint for addressing suicide—Awareness, Intervention, and Methodology, or AIM—an approach derived from the collaborative deliberations of the conference participants. As a framework for suicide prevention, AIM includes 15 key recommendations that were refined from consensus and evidence-based findings presented at the Reno conference. Recognizing that mental and substance abuse disorders confer the greatest risk for suicidal behavior, these recommendations suggest an important approach to preventing suicide and injuries from suicidal behavior by addressing the problems of undetected and undertreated mental and substance abuse disorders in conjunction with other public health approaches.

These recommendations and their supporting conceptual framework are essential steps toward a comprehensive National Strategy for Suicide Prevention. Other necessary elements will include constructive public health policy, measurable overall objectives, ways to monitor and evaluate progress toward these objectives, and provision of resources for groups and agencies identified to carry out the recommendations. The nation needs to move forward with these crucial recommendations and support continued efforts to improve the scientific bases of suicide prevention.

Many people, from public health leaders and mental and substance abuse disorder health experts to community advocates and suicide survivors, worked together in developing and proposing AIM for the American public. AIM and its recommendations chart a course for suicide prevention action now as well as serve as the foundation for a more comprehensive National Strategy for Suicide Prevention in the future. Together, they represent a critical component of a broader initiative to improve the mental health of the nation. I endorse the ongoing work necessary to complete a National Strategy because I believe that such a coordinated and evidence-based approach is the best way to use our resources to prevent suicide in America.

But even the most well-considered plan accomplishes nothing if it is not implemented. To translate AIM into action, each of us, whether we play a role at the federal, state, or local level, must turn these recommendations into programs best suited for our own communities. We must act now. We cannot change the past, but together we can shape a different future.

David Satcher, M.D., Ph.D.
Assistant Secretary for Health and Surgeon General

*Source:* US Public Health Service. (1999). *The Surgeon General's call to action to prevent suicide.* Washington, D.C.: Dept. of Health & Human Services.
http://www.surgeongeneral.gov/library/calltoaction/calltoaction.htm

# PREVENTION

For young people 15-24 years old, suicide is the third leading cause of death, behind unintentional injury and homicide (CDC, National Center of Injury Prevention Control). The *Surgeon General's Call To Action* introduces an outline for preventing suicide (see Figure 3-2) that prompted action throughout the United States. Prevention can take many forms. Knowledge of suicidal signs is essential in suicide prevention, particularly for the health professional. Paracetamol® (acetaminophen) is a drug frequently used in intentional overdoses. Prevention efforts may target an entire community or an individual. Prevention includes depression screenings, public information campaigns that encourage a healthy lifestyle, and efforts to educate physicians and other health care providers in signs of depression and suicide risk factors (Fiske & Abore, 2000-2001).

## Public Health Strategies

The first step in suicide prevention begins with defining the problem. Information is gathered about the characteristics of suicidal persons, incidents and events that precipitate suicidal acts, and support that makes a difference. The second step identifies causes, risk factors, and groups of people at risk. It also identifies protective factors that can prevent suicide (see Table 3-3). The third step is developing and testing interventions, and testing the effectiveness of each approach. The fourth step is implementing interventions that have demonstrated effectiveness in preventing suicide and suicidal behavior (US Public Health Service [USPHS], 1999).

## The Surgeon General's Call To Action

The *Surgeon General's Call To Action* introduces a blueprint for addressing suicide—Awareness, Intervention, and Methodology (AIM). AIM includes 15 key recommendations and serves as a framework for immediate action (see Table 3-4). The Surgeon General noted the significance of pro-

| TABLE 3-3: PROTECTIVE FACTORS |
|---|
| • Effective and appropriate clinical care for mental, physical, and substance abuse disorders |
| • Easy access to a variety of clinical interventions and support for help seeking |
| • Restricted access to highly lethal methods of suicide |
| • Family and community support |
| • Support from ongoing medical and mental health care relationships |
| • Learned skills in problem solving, conflict resolution, and nonviolent handling of disputes |
| • Cultural and religious beliefs that discourage suicide and support self-preservation instincts |
| *Source:* US Public Health Service. (1999). *The Surgeon General's call to action to prevent suicide.* Washington, D.C.: Dept. of Health & Human Services. http://www.surgeongeneral.gov/library/calltoaction/calltoaction.htm |

moting a public/private collaboration with the media, which affects our attitudes and influences our behavior (USPHS, 1999).

## Suicide and the Media

Media researchers are in general agreement that individuals are influenced by a variety of circumstances, from reading newspapers to discussion (Coleman, 1993). Research on a relationship between media and suicide has been documented. A study (Martin, 1998) supports the association between media coverage and increased suicide. Suicide covered in print media such as newspaper stories has been shown to increase imitative suicide behaviors. U.S. suicide statistics were compared with suicides that appeared on the front page of the New York Times from 1948 through 1968. Monthly suicides significantly increased. This study suggests that the rate of suicide imitation increases when pictures were included in the reporting. If the stories were extensive and if the word *suicide* was in a large headline, there was greater frequency of imitative behavior.

The significance of imitative suicidal behavior is so great that the *Werther effect* has become an accepted term to describe the action (Phillips, 1979; Etzersdorfer & Sonneck, 1998; Martin, 1998). The

## TABLE 3-4: AWARENESS, INTERVENTION, AND METHODOLOGY

**Awareness: Appropriately broaden the public's awareness of suicide and its risk factors**

1.  Promote public awareness that suicide is a public health problem and, as such, many suicides are preventable. Use information technology appropriately to make facts about suicide and its risk factors and prevention approaches available to the public and to health care providers.

2.  Expand awareness of and enhance resources in communities for suicide prevention programs and mental and substance abuse disorder assessment and treatment.

3.  Develop and implement strategies to reduce the stigma associated with mental illness, substance abuse, and suicidal behavior and with seeking help for such problems.

**Intervention: Enhance services and programs, both population-based and clinical care**

4.  Extend collaboration with and among public and private sectors to complete a National strategy for Suicide Prevention.

5.  Improve the ability of primary care providers to recognize and treat depression, substance abuse, and other major mental illnesses associated with suicide risk. Increase the referral to specialty care when appropriate.

6.  Eliminate barriers in public and private insurance programs for provision of quality mental and substance abuse disorder treatments and create incentives to treat patients with coexisting mental and substance abuse disorders.

7.  Institute training for all health, mental health, substance abuse and human service professionals (including clergy, teachers, correctional workers, and social workers) concerning suicide risk assessment and recognition, treatment, management, and aftercare interventions.

8.  Develop and implement effective training programs for family members of those at risk and for natural community helpers on how to recognize, respond to, and refer people showing signs of suicide risk and associated mental and substance abuse disorders. Natural community helpers are people such as educators, coaches, hairdressers, and faith leaders, among others.

9.  Develop and implement safe and effective programs in educational settings for youth that address adolescent distress, provide crisis intervention and incorporate peer support for seeking help.

10. Enhance community care resources by increasing the use of schools and workplaces as access and referral points for mental and physical health services and substance abuse treatment programs and provide support for persons who survive the suicide of someone close to them.

11. Promote a public/private collaboration with the media to assure that entertainment and news coverage represent balanced and informed portrayals of suicide and its associated risk factors including mental illness and substance abuse disorders and approaches to prevention and treatment.

**Methodology: Advance the science of suicide prevention**

12. Enhance research to understand risk and protective factors related to suicide, their interaction, and their effects on suicide and suicidal behaviors. Additionally, increase research on effective suicide prevention programs, clinical treatments for suicidal individuals, and culture-specific interventions.

13. Develop additional scientific strategies for evaluating suicide prevention interventions and ensure that evaluation components are included in all suicide prevention programs.

14. Establish mechanisms for federal, regional, and state interagency public health collaboration toward improving monitoring systems for suicide and suicidal behaviors and develop and promote standard terminology in these systems.

15. Encourage the development and evaluation of new prevention technologies, including firearm safety measures, to reduce easy access to lethal means of suicide.

*Source:* US Public Health Service. (1999). *The Surgeon General's call to action to prevent suicide.* Washington, D.C.: Dept. of Health & Human Services. http://www.surgeongeneral.gov/library/calltoaction/calltoaction.htm

concept of the Werther effect has its origin in Goethe's literary hero's suicide, whose act others imitated following his death. A study (Etzerdorfer & Sonneck, 1998) examined the imitation factor by creating a study group of the Austrian Association for Suicide Prevention. Since the installation of the subway, the rate of suicide was increasing, as people jumped in front of the oncoming trains. A press campaign was launched in 1987 that aimed to educate media on reporting suicides in a less dramatic way. The study was designed to collect and analyze the rate of suicides from that year.

Through this press campaign, journalists were informed about negative reporting of suicide and were given alternate ways of reporting that type of death. The journalists became better educated about reporting suicides of those who jumped in front of oncoming trains. As the media reporting of suicides changed, so did the rate of suicide. Suicide and attempted suicide fell more than 80% from the first to the second half of 1987 and the rate of suicide in Vienna remains at a low level.

Etzersdorfer and Sonneck (1998) maintain that there are ways to control the social impact of reported suicides if the following guidelines are in place:

The trigger-effect will be bigger, the more details of the special methods are reported, the more suicide is reported as being inconceivable ("he had everything life can give"), the more the motives are reported to be romantic ("to be forever united"), the more simplifications are used ("suicide because of bad news"). The attention will be bigger if the report is printed on the front page, if the term "suicide" is used in the headline, if there is a photograph of the person who committed suicide, if the attitude of the person is implicitly described as being heroic and desirable ("he had to do that in this situation"). The effect will be smaller if more alternatives are shown ("where is it possible to find help in such a situation?"), if there are reports about a crisis

that was overcome and did not result in suicide, if readers are provided with background information on suicide behavior and suicide in general (such as what to do with someone who expressed suicidal thoughts) (p. 69).

The investigators found a correlation between the more moderate reporting of suicide in the media and a decrease in suicides. Subway suicides were significantly reduced and remained at a low level. Their results indicted that by changing the reporting of suicides in the media, the suicide rate could be lowered.

A study of 49 hospitals in the United Kingdom found an association between suicide by poison on a television drama titled *Casualty* and a short-lived increase in imitation suicide attempts by poison. A 3-week period was studied following the drama and compared to a 3-week period before the drama (O'Connor et al., 1999). Of 1,047 completed questionnaires, 18% of overdose patients had seen the episode of *Casualty*. Compared to the 3-week period before the broadcast, self-poisoning increased by 17% the week following the broadcast. Self-poisoning increased by 9% the second week following the program. The television drama may have influenced those vulnerable, as 15% reported that viewing the episode had influenced their decision to take an overdose.

Of the 32 patients who survived their suicide attempt, 20% reported that the television drama influenced their behavior to attempt suicide and 17% imitated the ingestion of Paracetamol®, the same drug shown on the television drama. Although interesting, this is not statistically significant. However, Hawton's study provided us with the insight into how the broadcasting of dramas depicting self-poisoning may have a short-term influence in the rate of overdose and changes in the choice of drug taken by those vulnerable.

To determine whether viewing a fictional television film influences the viewer's attitudes and emotional response about suicide, a study was done on 119 non-suicidal college students (Biblarz, Biblarz,

Baldree, & Pilgram, 1991). The students were put into three groups. One group saw *Surviving,* a film about suicide. The second group saw *Death Wish,* which contained no overt suicidal images. The third group saw *That's Entertainment,* a musical without any aggression or suicidal images. Each student was given a questionnaire prior to watching the films. The exact questionnaire was administered immediately after the viewing and then again 2 weeks later. The study showed that there is a correlation between an increased emotional arousal score immediately after viewing the film and the film content. Only the students who viewed the films *Surviving* and *Death Wish* had increased arousal scores immediately after viewing the films. What is important to note is that this level of arousal was not maintained. The arousal for both groups decreased 2 weeks later to slightly below pre-film levels.

In a study on imitation and suggestion, it was found that just after publicized suicides, the rates of automobile fatalities increased (Phillips, 1979). The more publicity the story received, the higher the later automobile fatality rate. Interestingly enough, reports of younger suicides were followed by younger people dying by vehicle crashes and reports of older suicides were followed by older people dying by vehicle crashes. The author believes that the correlation between the reporting of the stories and the increase in suicide at that time might be a result of imitating, modeling, and suggestion by the drivers.

Phillips examined a 2-week period beginning 2 days prior to the publicized suicide and ending 11 days later. The researcher found that automobile fatalities increased by 31% in the 3 days after a suicide as reported in the media. There were no other variables involved in the increase in suicides, and the increase in the suicide rate wasn't due to the day of the week, monthly fluctuations in motor vehicle fatalities, holiday weekends, or to yearly linear trends (Phillips, 1979). It is also interesting to note that the

motor vehicle fatalities are most frequent in the region where the suicide story is publicized.

---

> ***Personal Insight***
> *Look at a current movie or television program, paying special attention to how death and or suicide are portrayed. Do you find that you are influenced by what you are seeing?*

---

## Population-Based Prevention

Population-based prevention strategies focus on at-risk groups, such as students, the elderly, those who are gay, those with a psychiatric illness, and alcoholics. One population-based prevention strategy for students at risk is no-suicide agreements. Rather than using therapy alone for suicidal adolescents, high school and college students held a positive view toward using no-suicide agreements as part of the treatment, although high school student's support of the agreements was lukewarm (Myers & Range, 2002).

Stuart, Waalen, and Haelstromm (2003) studied the efficacy of training peer helpers in suicide risk assessment in a comprehensive school-based suicide prevention program. The authors maintain that the prevention program must go beyond basic peer-helping and

> for peer helpers to be an effective component of a suicide prevention program, they not only need basic training in empathy and active listening, but they also need training in suicide risk assessment and encouragement to seek out the angry and isolated peers in their school and develop relationships with them even though those relationships might be resisted or difficult (p. 331).

Elderly people (65+ years) in the United States have a higher suicide rate than any other age group (see Figure 3-3). An average of 5,393 elderly people kill themselves annually in the United States, which means that 14.8 elderly people die by suicide each day. One elderly person completes suicide every 1 hour 37.5 minutes (American Association for

## FIGURE 3-3: OLDER ADULTS AND DEPRESSION

In a given year, between one and two percent of people over age 65 living in the community, i.e., not living in nursing homes or other institutions, suffer from major depression and about two percent have dysthymia. Depression, however, is not a normal part of aging. Research has clearly demonstrated the importance of diagnosing and treating depression in older persons. Because major depression is typically a recurrent disorder, relapse prevention is a high priority for treatment research. As noted previously, a recent NIMH-supported study established the efficacy of combined antidepressant medication and interpersonal psychotherapy in reducing depressive relapses in older adults who had recovered from an episode of depression.

Additionally, recent NIMH studies show that 13 to 27 percent of older adults have subclinical depressions that do not meet the diagnostic criteria for major depression or dysthymia but are associated with increased risk of major depression, physical disability, medical illness, and high use of health services. Subclinical depressions cause considerable suffering, and some clinicians are now beginning to recognize and treat them.

Suicide is more common among the elderly than in any other age group. NIMH research has shown that nearly all people who commit suicide have a diagnosable mental or substance abuse disorder. In studies of older adults who committed suicide, nearly all had major depression, typically a first episode, though very few had a substance abuse disorder. Suicide among white males aged 85 and older was nearly six times the national U.S. rate (65 per 100,000 compared with 11 per 100,000) in 1996, the most recent year for which statistics are available. Prevention of suicide in older adults is a high priority area in the NIMH prevention research portfolio.

*Source:* National Institute of Mental Health. (1999). Fact sheet: Depression research at the National Institute of Mental Health. Bethesda, MD: NIH. Publication No 00-4501. Reprinted 2000, updated 2002. http://www.nimh.nih.gov/publicat/depresfact.cfm

Suicidology). Geriatric suicide is differentiated by fewer warning signs, more lethal means of ending life, and greater incidences of depression and physical illness than suicide in children and adults. To better prevent suicide, there must be adequate understanding of the risk factors for the behavior or disorders that are being targeted (Pearson, 2000-2001). The Center for Elderly Suicide Prevention (CESP) seeks to prevent suicide in the elderly by identifying and addressing possible risk factors (e.g., social isolation, bereavement, depression) for suicide. CESP provides a 24-hour friendship line, individual counseling, friendly home visits, and psychotherapy home visits for seniors aged 60 and over.

When D'Augelli, Hershberger, and Pilkington (2001) studied suicidality patterns and sexual orientations of 350 lesbian, gay, and bisexual youths aged 14 to 21, they found that suicide attempts often occurred after the subjects became aware of their sexual feelings and before they told their parents or any one else of their sexual orientation. The authors

concluded that over a quarter of the adolescents sampled reported a suicide attempt in their family. The findings show that prevention should be sensitive to their unique needs, fostering family and social supports, while encouraging professional counseling.

Another population based strategy includes common treatment for schizophrenics. In the U.S., case management or individual psychotherapy with medication is probably the most common treatment for schizophrenia (Fenton, 2000). Few studies show the benefit of psychiatric treatment, possibly due to methodological problems. Dorwart and Ostacher (1999) point out that:

The problem in documenting that psychiatric treatment can reduce suicide risk should not discourage efforts to prevent suicide but instead call forth a doubling of our efforts to do so. The limitations of specific treatment systems can approach the problem of treating potentially suicidal patients. If these were to be studied, we would probably find that they have significant effects on the outcomes for such patients (p. 59).

Drinking within 3 hours of the suicide attempt was associated with nearly lethal attempts. Roy (2001) notes strategies to treat alcoholism include Alcoholics Anonymous (AA) meetings, prescribing naltrexone and acamprosate as aids in prolonging abstinence from alcohol, and treating comorbid depression.

Having population-based prevention strategies in place for students, the elderly, people of alternate sexual orientation, alcoholics, and those with a psychiatric illness is a worthy approach for reaching out to those in high-risk groups. Other special populations at risk include Native Americans, some Asian-Americans, young white males, and Hispanic students (see Table 3-5). The group that has the lowest suicide rate in America is African-American women, who may possess defenses such as their culture, religion, and social support, along with a negative attitude toward suicide (Marion & Range, 2003). The authors found that African-American women reported suicide as an unacceptable act. Perhaps if this attitude toward suicide reaches into other populations, the strategy can be adopted and suicide more widely prevented.

## Prevention in Primary Care

Interventions in primary care settings and community outreach to isolated and at-risk elderly individuals are two recommended approaches in preventing geriatric suicide (Conwell, 2001). Suicidal older adults rarely seek out mental health services. They are more likely to go to their primary care physician for support than a mental health provider as shown in the following example.

### Example

It appeared a routine Monday afternoon at a general practitioner's office. Yet shortly after 1pm, an elderly patient arrived for his appointment. Through the years, he had always greeted the nurse with a warm hello. However, today he walked slow-

---

### TABLE 3-5: AT A GLANCE: SUICIDE AMONG SPECIAL POPULATIONS

- During the period from 1979-1992, suicide rates for Native Americans (a category that includes American Indians and Alaska Natives) were about 1.5 times the national rates. There were a disproportionate number of suicides among young male Native Americans during this period, as males 15-24 accounted for 64% of all suicides by Native Americans.

- Suicide rates are higher than the national average for some groups of Asian Americans. For example, the suicide rate among Asian Americans and Pacific Islanders in the state of California is similar to that of the total population. However, in Hawaii the rate for AAPI's jumps to 11.2 per 100,000 people, compared to 10.8 per 100,000 rate for all people residing there. Asian-American women have the highest suicide rate among women 65 or older.

- While the suicide rate among young people is greatest among young white males, from 1980 through 1996 the rate increased most rapidly among black males aged 15 to 19—more than doubling from 3.6 per 100,000 to 8.1 per 100,000

- In a survey of students in 151 high schools around the country, the 1997 Youth Risk Behavior Surveillance System found that Hispanic students (10.7%) were significantly more likely than white students (6.3%) to have reported a suicide attempt. Among Hispanic students, females (14.9%) were more than twice as likely as males (7.2%) to have reported a suicide attempt. But Hispanic male students (7.2%) were significantly more likely than white male students (3.2%) to report this behavior.

*Source:*US Public Health Service. (1999). *The Surgeon General's call to action to prevent suicide.* Washington, D.C.: Dept. of Health & Human Services. http://www.surgeongeneral.gov/library/calltoaction/fact7.htm

---

ly to the examination room. Usually very alert and talkative, today he seemed lost in his own thoughts. The nurse asked him how he was feeling and he whispered, "I'm fine." She asked if he was feeling unhappy lately. He told her that all his friends were gone. He said, "They are all dead." She was empathetic and mentioned how difficult that must be for him. He said, "I am all alone now. Nobody needs me. I don't know why I keep waking up every morning." She asked, "Do you ever hope that you go to sleep and not wake up?" He said that he was having those thoughts. She asked, "Are you thinking about suicide?" He said, "It has been on my mind lately, and I can't seem to get the idea out of my head." The physician walked into the room and asked how he was doing. He said, "I am fine." The nurse shared with the physician their conversation. The doctor then explored the patient's loneliness and suicide ideation.

Hopelessness, depression, physical illness, and access to a gun can lead to geriatric suicide. It may be difficult to assess older clients, who are more inclined to kill themselves when suicidal thoughts arise, because they are less inclined to reveal their suicidal intentions than younger age groups (Miller, Segal, & Coolidge, 2001). Miller et al. found that religious beliefs and having children were a stronger reason for older adults not to complete suicide. These moral objections were reasons why the adults chose not to end their life.

Primary care physicians play an integral role in suicide prevention as they detect and treat mental disorders and substance abuse disorders (Dorwart & Ostacher, 1999). White elderly males are more at risk (Hughes & Kleespies, 2001). Most individuals who are medically ill do not have an increased risk of suicide. However, some physical illnesses associated with mental or substance abuse can increase the risk for suicide (AIDS, cancer of the brain, and multiple sclerosis).

# INTERVENTION

## Assessing Suicidal Behaviors

In 2001, suicide is the eleventh ranking cause of death in the U.S. and is a serious health problem caused by an interaction of psychological, biological, and sociological factors. The very concept of

intervention implies an involvement with an individual to avert the suicide. Nurses can help avert the suicide, but they must be prepared for the task at hand. The American Association of Suicidology recommends some ways to be helpful to someone who is threatening suicide.

- Be direct. Talk openly and matter-of-factly about suicide.

- Be willing to listen. Allow expressions of feelings. Accept the feelings.

- Be non-judgmental. Don't debate whether suicide is right or wrong or whether feelings are good or bad. Don't lecture on the value of life.

- Get involved. Become available. Show interest and support.

- Don't dare him or her to do it.

- Don't act shocked. This will put distance between you.

- Don't be sworn to secrecy. Seek support.

- Offer hope that alternatives are available but do not offer glib reassurance.

- Take action. Remove means, such as guns or stockpiled pills.

- Get help from persons or agencies specializing in crisis intervention and suicide prevention (American Association of Suicidology).

Health professionals may feel anxious or unprepared when working with suicidal patients due to their level of training and experience. A professional's attitudes toward suicide, their own history of suicidality, and death acceptance are all factors that relate to suicide intervention competencies (Neimeyer, Fortner, & Melby, 2001). A good strategy for intervention is knowing which mental health professional or provider to contact when someone is in a suicidal crisis. *Psychiatrists* are medical doctors trained to specialize in mental disorders, they can prescribe drugs. They look at emotional problems as illnesses and may have admitting privileges at local hospitals. *Mental health counselors* have extensive schooling and training in dealing with problems in individual and group therapy.

Other mental health professionals are *psychologists*. They treat individuals by using psychological techniques but do not prescribe drugs. If necessary, they refer to healthcare practitioners for medicatable disorders that are caused by abnormal brain chemistry. Mental health professionals receive years of training and many states require licensure. *Clinical social workers* have at least a master's degree in social work (M.S.W.) and 2 years of experience in a clinical setting. Social workers counsel those with emotional problems and also arrange for needed social services. *Psychiatric nurse-specialists* are nurses who are certified to work in psychiatric settings. *Psychoanalysts* are psychiatrists or psychologists with special training in psychoanalysis. This approach involves intense exploration of the patient's unconscious mind in order for patients to remember early traumas that have been blocked. Whoever provides professional intervention, it is crucial that the environment will enable the individual to feel most comfortable and will support a rapport leading to an effective evaluation of the severity of suicide ideation.

When assessing for suicide ideation, the initial assessment involves looking at imminent risk. The presence of risk factors is a signal for the provider that the patient needs help. Depending upon the acute risk, hospitalization may be necessary. Phrases such as *"I wish I were dead"* or *"I'm going to end it all"* are verbal clues that an individual may be suicidal. Phrases such as *"What's the point of going on?"* or *"You would be better off without me,"* and *"I can't go on anymore"* are phrases that are not as direct, but they still may be a clue to suicide ideation.

Looking at the lethality of the plan, the professional evaluates the intent, behaviors, and predictable consequences of that behavior. Certain behaviors can include purchasing a gun, giving away possessions, or putting personal and business

affairs in order. Additionally, individuals who have suffered from depression and suddenly exhibit behavior of elation are also considered high risk. This time following a depression can be considered a vulnerable one, for it is at this time that many individuals complete suicide. Therefore, someone considered at risk should be monitored for months following a depression.

In assessing and treating suicide behaviors, we need to look at the most common methods of suicide. Men often use more violent means such as guns or hanging, and women more often use drugs or carbon monoxide poisoning (Denning, Conwell, King, & Cox, 2000). The most common method of suicide in the United States is by firearm. It is estimated that 16,869 men and women die annually by firearm suicide, and 6,198 individuals die by suffocation/hanging (American Association for Suicidology, 2003).

A health professional looks at predisposing conditions, including the link between those factors and the desire to end life. As coping skills are discussed, the focus should remain on the individual, and interruptions should be avoided. Jacobs, Brewer, and Klein-Benheim (1999) point out several questions regarding suicidal thoughts to ask a patient when gauging the severity of their suicidal ideation:

- Have you had thoughts about harming yourself?
- What are the thoughts?
- When did they begin?
- How frequent are they?
- How persistent are they?
- Are they obsessive?
- Can you control them?
- Are there command hallucinations?

When managing a suicidal patient, the professional should continuously monitor the lethality of the plan, consult with a peer, hospitalize the patient if necessary, show personal concern, involve significant others in the patient's life, and carefully modify the issue of confidentiality so that it is understood that statements regarding suicide will not be treated as a secret between patient and professional (Schneidman, 1993). Patients with psychiatric disorders benefit from clinical care intervention treatments. Roy (2001) notes that the interventions:

(a) reduce suicidal ideation or attempts;

(b) reduce impulsivity, anger, and self-directed aggression;

(c) improve compliance with treatment and medication-taking;

(d) reduce clinical symptoms or course features associated with suicide risk (e.g., recurrence of illness);

(e) treat comorbid disorders;

(f) arrange community supports and continuity of care during the post-discharge period;

(g) and educate physicians about the recognition and treatment of depression and how to assess suicide risk

(p. 69).

The National Institute of Mental Health has made recommendations regarding diagnostic evaluation for depression. The physician should take a comprehensive history of the severity of symptoms, when they began, and how long they have lasted. The history takes account of the patient's past symptoms and treatment. Questions asked include alcohol, drug use, and suicide ideation, family history of depression, treatment, and effectiveness. The physician can also perform a mental status examination to establish if speech, thoughts, or memory has been affected (NIMH, 2003).

---

*Personal Insight*
*Suppose a co-worker or patient was suicidal. What would you do?*

---

# ASSISTED SUICIDE AND EUTHANASIA

Euthanasia is derived from the Greek words *eu,* meaning "good," and *thanatos,* meaning "death." Euthanasia is the active form of mercy killing. There are two forms of euthanasia, active euthanasia and passive. Active euthanasia is otherwise known as assisted suicide or assisted death, in which an act is committed. The patient administers a death-causing agent to end his or her life with the assistance of someone who provides the means, typically a physician. The second type of euthanasia, passive euthanasia, involves omission of an act. The physician may withhold oxygen, antibiotics, or intravenous feedings from those who are terminally ill.

Physician-assisted suicide occurs when the physician provides the means, such as giving the patient information on how to end their life, prescribing medication, or giving the patient equipment. Rubel (1999a) maintains, "All too often patients ask their physicians to help them die when what they really are asking for is to help them live without pain" (p. 326). Those in favor of euthanasia believe that an individual should not die in unbearable pain and suffering (Street & Kissane, 1999-2000).

Voluntary active euthanasia is when a clearly competent patient makes a voluntary request of a physician to administer a lethal dose of medication to end the patient's life. This requests an aid in dying. To address concerns about attitudes toward legalization of active voluntary euthanasia (AVE) and physician-assisted suicide (PAS), Dickinson, Lancaster, Clark, Ahmedzai, & Noble (2002) found that

Physicians were in overwhelming agreement on the following: The patient should be mentally competent; the physician should have an established relationship with the patient; two physicians should be in accord with the decision; and a specific waiting period after the request should be in place (p. 485).

*Discussed assisted suicide* is defined as the physician discussing alternatives, encouraging the individual to look at all options. *Encouraged assisted suicide* is where the physician encourages the suicide and may provide the means to end the individual's life. Werth (2000) notes the major arguments against assisted death. People who want assisted death:

1. are committing suicide;

2. are suffering from a mental illness, probably clinical depression;

3. could do it themselves, so asking for assistance is a "cry for help;"

4. have not considered other alternatives;

5. are being pressured by unscrupulous or overwhelmed significant others;

6. are doing so due to pressure from medical service providers;

7. are suffering from the internalization of negative societal attitudes.

In addition, assisted death:

8. will have a negative impact on significant others;

9. will lead to a societal devaluation of life for particular classes of people;

10. cannot be regulated and therefore an ever-increasing group of people will be killed. Although these mental health-related arguments against assisted death are made in almost every forum, all of them can also be made, at least to some degree, against withholding/withdrawing treatment

(p. 260).

One of the questions asked on Worthen and Yeatts' (2000-2001) survey instrument was, "If a person is slowly dying with a painful disease that cannot be cured, should a physician be allowed to assist the patient to end his or her life, if that's the patient's wish?" (p. 132). Though age, gender, and level of care for terminally ill loved ones were not significant factors affecting attitudes toward assisted suicide, individuals who were more religious, with the belief that life belongs to God, were least likely to seek assisted suicide. These individuals viewed assisted suicide as murder (Worthen & Yeatts, 2000-2001).

The National Hospice Organization is opposed to physician-assisted suicide. Mesler & Miller (2000) maintain, "The hospice philosophy is to make terminal patients as comfortable as possible—physically, psychically, socially, and spiritually, while neither hastening nor postponing death" (p. 135). Margaret, an Eastern Hope nurse with 5 years of experience, maintains:

> I find it hard at times working here, hard with what I see; working with these young people who are dying, and watching the transition unfold...starting to fall, lost many of their faculties, lose bowel and bladder control, and the confusion. It's terribly hard to see. It's terribly hard for the families... And it (assisted suicide) seems a very logical, rational, sensible, right choice. And I can understand somebody choosing it. Yet I don't—maybe it's my own personal faith in God, religious philosophy, beliefs, my own experience of suffering — but I feel that there is meaning behind it [the dying process] (Mesler & Miller, p. 150).

There is a biological link between depression and suicide. A considerable number of those who are chronically and terminally ill, especially those who express an interest in assisted suicide, are clinically depressed. Werth (2000) maintains that it is it is not easy to diagnose the depression because symptoms of depression have common characteristics with symptoms related to the disease or treatments for the disease. Medically ill patients may want to die because they do not want to live the rest of their life in a deteriorating condition. In describing rational suicide, Siegel (1986) stated:

> The defining characteristics of a rational suicide are: (1) the individual possesses a

realistic assessment of his [or her] situation, (2) the mental processes leading to his [or her] decision to commit suicide are unimpaired by psychological illness or severe emotional distress, and (3) the motivational basis of his [or her] decision would be understandable to the majority of uninvolved observers from his [or her] community or social group (p. 407).

The experience of suffering makes the individual feel hopeless, which could lead to suicide ideation as shown in the following example.

### Example

A thirty-two-year old woman, diagnosed with cancer, presented to the ER with severe nausea and abdominal pain. Her husband brought her in to the ER; however, she does not want any further medical intervention. Knowing she is terminal, she informs the nurse that she has contemplated suicide. As a medically ill patient, she felt that she would rather die by suicide than die by cancer. Her nurse recommends a psychiatric evaluation even though she believes that it is a rational choice for her to want to shorten the period of time she would be dying.

Suffering can be caused by mental anguish or physical pain. Rubel (1999a) notes,

When physicians in our society alleviate pain, they fill the individual's landscape with hope. That hope stems from the knowledge that the physician has effectively reduced suffering. Physicians who can alleviate pain offer their patients a meaningful existence through good medicine, whether they are terminally ill or have many years of life ahead of them. There is hope that the patients' lives will end naturally, and not by their own hand or that of their physician (p. 331).

## Physician-Assisted Suicide and the Dying Patient

What choices do the terminally ill have as they face their greatest battle, and why does it become a struggle in the first place? The battle comes when the needs of the terminally ill are not met. The terminally ill fight this battle when they are forced to deal with emotional or physical pain. Harrold (1998) explains that patients and family are afraid that the terminally ill will become addicted to the pain medications due to side effects of medicines. Most feel the pain medications should be given only when pain is so severe that it cannot be tolerated. The research clearly shows that as the terminally ill struggle with such issues, their physicians and nurses struggle with their own. Physicians fear legislative or regulatory action if they prescribe opioids in the dosages required for pain control (Harrold, 1998). Though the terminally ill fight the battle and endure the suffering, there are no winners in this war.

Shneidman (1993) maintains that

physicians and other health professionals need the courage and wisdom to work on a person's suffering at a phenomenological level and to explore such questions as "How do you hurt?" and "How may I help you?" They should then do whatever is necessary, using a wide variety of legitimate tactics...to reduce that person's self-destructive impulses.

Peace is found when the self-destructive impulses are managed appropriately. With this understanding, nurses, social workers, and psychologists can work as a team to help the patient and family through the crisis. Palliative care should be discussed, as the terminally ill fear suffering and dying in unremitting pain. Hendin (1998) explains that:

we now know that giving analgesic medicine to patients at regular intervals rather than waiting for their pain to intensify provides better relief for chronic pain. Even our recent discovery that antidepressant medication can be effective in relieving otherwise intractable pain suggests the complexity of the perception of pain (p. 235).

Gilbar and Cohen (1995) report that Israeli oncologists, when treating cancer patients, must share details of the patient's care and assist them in voicing their concerns and opinions. Cancer patients may need help to articulate their wants and desires. What they need is an end to their physical and emotional suffering. The end can involve compassionate care rather than physician-assisted suicide, and physicians must be reimbursed for providing that care. Insufficient reimbursement for end-of-life care is a concern of physicians (Harrold, 1998). This can include services that may not be reimbursed or are simply too expensive for the patient and their family member.

One problem facing the terminally ill is their suicide ideation. The nurse should intervene if the patient is suicidal. The intervention itself is to discuss all options. If the patient is defining those options as suicidal ones, then exploring why they are thinking about those options is appropriate. Nurses should alert other trained professionals that their terminally ill patient is exhibiting suicide ideation. Werth (1999) writes:

Turning to the ethics codes of the different national mental health organizations, there is a lack of agreement over the ethical obligations of members of the respective groups in situations involving potential harm to self. The American Psychiatric Association (1995) stated (section 4, number 8) that "When...the risk of danger is deemed to be significant, the psychiatrist may reveal confidential information disclosed by the patient" (p. 6). Similarly, the APA (1992) indicated that "Psychologists disclose confidential information without the consent of the individual only as mandated by law, or where permitted by law, such as...to protect

the patient or client or others from harm" (p. 1606). Thus, these two organizations allow breaking of confidentiality but do not ethically require it (p. 243).

Nurses and other health professionals are responsible for managing the self-destructive impulses of their patients. Gostin (1997) maintains the importance of high quality end-of-life care with physical and mental pain management and the alleviation of depression. It is vital that nurses listen openly to suicidal patients and help them discover all the underlying issues, ranging from loss of dignity through spiritual needs to the fear of death. However, nurses sometimes create a safe emotional distance from their patients, which may contribute to the terminally ill falling deeper into depression and electing to end their life rather than be a burden on their family and health professionals.

As terminally ill individuals communicate their issues, nurses help them cope by discussing options. Hendin (1998) writes that physicians should "assure them that he or she will remain with them to the end and relieve their suffering" (p. 242). The nurse should reassure the patient that all the necessary measures will be taken as their condition worsens.

Oregon's experience with physician assisted suicide (PAS) is reported by Chin, Hedberg, Higginson, and Fleming (1999). The first year's experience (1998) shows some terminally ill Oregonians request PAS because they fear both emotional and physical suffering. Autonomy becomes a critical issue, when patients believe that they will be unable to participate in activities, lose control of bodily functions, and become a burden to family, friends, and caregivers. PAS is not an autonomous act on the part of the terminally ill, as the patient relinquishes control to the physician and gives the physician the right to end his or her suffering on the physician's terms. If pain and suffering were relieved first, PAS might not then be an option and the patient would be truly autonomous.

As the terminally ill struggle with end-of-life issues, they often endeavor to maintain a sense of self-determination while relinquishing elements of control to their caregiver. Some terminally ill people believe that they have the right to decide the manner in which they die. They may not want their family to be present as their bodies deteriorate. They do not want to experience the loss of bodily control. They do not want to go through the process of becoming a physical burden to their caregivers. Often they fear the physical pain caused by their illness.

If these patients receive counseling and are assured their needs will be met, they may not choose PAS. Brock, Holmes, Foley, and Homes (1992) and Foley, Miles, Brock, and Philips (1995) studied 1,227 elderly deaths. The caregivers reported that 33% were in pain during the last 24 hours before their death.

Physicians should treat the terminally ill fairly and provide them with the necessary pain medications. The terminally ill require their physicians to listen to their concerns and fears as they are communicated. The concerns and fears often include pain and personal image, particularly as they grow weaker and notice dramatic physical changes in themselves, loss of bodily functions, unfinished business, the need to remain in control of their treatment decisions, and access to the truth.

Many mental health professionals consider that people can make rational decisions to die and that talking about assisted death with clients could be an acceptable practice (Werth, 1999). The practice of discussing PAS and following through with completion of the act became a legal option for terminally ill Oregon residents on October 27, 1997.

The process includes making two verbal requests to a licensed Oregon physician 15 days apart and one written request. The Department of Human Resources (DHR), Oregon Health Division, reports that the terminally ill capable Oregon resident who is 18 years of age or older can obtain a prescription from his or her physician for lethal medications after 48 hours (Chin et al., 1999). A patient who is capable in the opinion of the court or the physician, psychiatrist, or psychologist, has the ability to make and communicate health care decisions to health care providers and individuals who know the way in which the patient communicates. If the patient is considered capable, the physician could then prescribe the medication that would end the person's life.

Adequate end-of-life care must be assured and must include treating underlying depression along with pain management. The suffering of the terminally ill can often be relieved by palliative care. In the very end of life, terminal sedation may be an option for those whose pain is unbearable. However, some health professionals believe that they are helping a patient die when administering the morphine drip, instead of asserting that they are managing pain in the end of life. Thomas Preston, a cardiologist, writing an Op-Ed piece for the New York Times (1994) writes, "It is given ostensibly to relieve pain, but over a period of time it can kill by depressing respiration . . . often the morphine drip is given with the real intention of killing the patient." The doctrine of double effect is that by aggressive palliation the pain can be relieved but the death is also hastened. The physician does not set out to murder his patient intentionally. The ethical distinction here is that the desired outcome is to stop the suffering in the very end of life, when there are no options left, and not to kill the patient, as Dr. Preston postulates.

A review of the literature reveals that the terminally ill who die by PAS are suffering in what they believe to be a helpless and hopeless situation. The Oregon Health Council formed Oregon Health Decisions (OHD) as an outreach program to conduct community meetings throughout Oregon to collect residents' views on bioethics and values, and look at the issues facing the terminally ill. The findings of the OHD have shown that autonomy and personal control are issues facing the terminally ill. Physicians must offer them hope that their pain will not be ignored, that their stress and psychological concerns will be treated appropriately, and that they will be cared for in a dignified manner, though they may lose control of bodily functions.

# POSTVENTION

Schneidman (1993) coined the term *postvention* as "those things done after the dire event has occurred that serve to mollify the after-effects of the event in a person who has attempted suicide, or to deal with the adverse effects as the survivor-victims of a person who has committed suicide." Suicide survivors are the family, friends, and significant others of those who completed suicide.

## Suicide Survivor Grief

*Be patient with everything unresolved in your heart and*
*Try to love the questions themselves...*
*Do not now seek the answers, which cannot be given to you now,*
*Because you would not be able to live them.*
*And the point is to live everything.*
*Live the questions now.*
*Perhaps then, someday far in the future,*
*You will gradually, without even noticing it,*
*Live your way into the answer.*

— Rainer Maria Rilke

Suicide survivor grief encompasses emotional, mental, social, spiritual, and intellectual dimensions. Barrett and Scott (1989) found four grief reactions unique to suicide survivors.

1. Those that normally result from the death of a family member, irrespective of the cause along with somatic symptoms, sense of hopelessness, feelings of anger and guilt, a loss of social support, and an increase in self-destructive tendencies.

2. Those that usually arise from a death whose cause is deemed not to be natural and is perceived as avoidable, including feelings of being stigmatized, abandoned, and shamed by the death.

3. Those that usually arise from an unanticipated death despite the cause including shock, search for an explanation of the death, feeling responsible and blamed.

4. Those that result from the additional trauma of dealing with the suicidal nature of the death, including feelings of rejection.

While providing help to suicide survivors, health professionals may be called upon to answer some difficult questions. Why did their loved one take their own life? When responding to the question, one must realize that there may never be an answer. It is most important to simply be able to explore the questions openly and honestly until the survivors find meaning in their loved one's life and death. Suicidal deaths are often sudden, and survivors have little if any chance to say goodbye. Most survivors are surprised by the news and then must adjust to a loss that was unnatural in many ways. Survivors may feel shame as they tell their friends, co-workers, and neighbors what happened. Survivors may experience guilt, anger, blame, and stigma as they cope with the loss.

McIntosh (1993) suggested four generalizations about suicide survivors.

(a) There appear to be more similarities than differences between suicide and other types of survivors (particularly sudden-death survivors).

(b) There may be a small number of grief reactions that are different for survivors, but there are not yet clearly established.

(c) The course of suicide bereavement may differ over time.

(d) After the second year, the reactions observed in suicide bereavement seem to show few differences from the mourning trajectory for other types of losses.

The mourning experience for survivors is unusual, as it may elevate their own suicidal risk factors due to the disruption in attachment, any substance abuse involved, or genetic predispositions such as depression and bipolar disorder. Family members may exhibit the suicidal behavior, believing that it is an acceptable way to end their pain (Jordan, 2001). Best predictors of reduced general health and post-traumatic distress for suicide survivors are isolation, little education, short time elapsed since the death, and female gender. Variables predicting complicated grief reactions for survivors are self-isolation, female gender, and lack of other children (Dyregrov, Nordanger, & Dyregrov, 2003).

One predominant shared feeling is shame. The shame felt derives from a history of stigma. Rubel (1999b) notes,

> to understand the grief response of suicide survivors, one has to explore how society has treated them historically. The issues related to their type of grief come from a history of shame and social outcast. In 18th century Europe, the suicide victim's body was dragged through the streets. Some were decapitated, thrown to wild beasts, or hung upside down. The body, denied a proper burial, would usually be placed in a sewer or brought to the side of the road, maybe with a stake through its heart, and covered with stones. In addition, survivors were forced to leave their homes, leaving behind all their goods and property (p. 8).

With a history of shame and social stigma, survivors reach out to those who will provide support. Survivors will explore their perception of the event, what preceded the act, and with whom their loved one came in contact with before killing themselves. Often they will seek out clinicians who were working with their loved ones.

The aim of a recent study consisting of 71 suicide survivors was to examine their perceptions of clinicians who were treating their loved one at the time of their death. Survivors reported what was most helpful after the death in regard to the clinician's behavior. Of the survivors, 21% reported the

clinician making contact, 17% found the clinician offering his/her condolences, and 15% reported their clinician discussing his/her experience and sense of loss to be most helpful to them and their family. Of the 71 survivors, 23% felt that the clinician made a mistake regarding medication decisions and 27% reported their attitudes and/or beliefs toward mental health care had changed, now including a lack of faith in the clinician's mental health care system.

Since 12 clinicians lose a patient to suicide each week in the United States, the results indicated that clinicians must manage their own grief as well as the grief of the survivors. The study has produced evidence that clinicians must be mindful to contact the family of the victim by phone or face-to-face meetings. When clinician made contact and were straightforward and open, the survivors were less likely to bring a lawsuit against them (Peterson, Luoma, & Dunne, 2002).

> **_Personal Insight_**
>
> Have you ever known anyone who completed suicide? If so, in what ways did the suicide survivors find comfort and support? Knowing what you do now, what recommendations would you make to them?

## Suicide Survivor Support Groups

Suicide survivor support groups bring together individuals who have experienced the suicidal death of a family member, friend, or significant other. Survivors share their feelings and thoughts openly and honestly among others who have experienced similar losses. Common statements made by group members include "No one mentions his name," and "I haven't told anyone the truth about how he died." Guilt is another common feeling among suicide survivors. Survivors often believe that they could have done something to prevent the suicide. Blame is a common bond among survivors of suicide. Survivors may need to find someone to blame for the suicide (i.e. the doctor, therapist, family members, friends, themselves, as well as the victim). The suicide survivor group gives them the opportunity to ask questions and focus on their most pressing issues and concerns.

# SUMMARY

This chapter examined suicide and life-threatening behavior. The chapter began by defining suicide and identifying the psychological, biological, and sociological explanations of suicide. Emile Durkheim's study of suicide in 1897 concluded that the social suicide rate was determined by the degree of social integration and the degree of social regulation. A number of terms relevant to understanding suicide, such as altruistic, egotistic, fatalistic, and anomic suicides, were identified.

The next part of this chapter examined the *Surgeon General's Call To Action* to prevent suicide. We noted the signs and symptoms of suicide, public health strategies in prevention, and the significance of imitative suicidal behavior and the reporting of suicide in the media. Population-based prevention strategies among students, the elderly, those who are gay, those with a psychiatric illness, and addicts were highlighted. Prevention in primary care settings, community outreach, intervention, and assessment of suicidal behaviors was discussed. In this chapter, the roles of the psychologist, clinical social worker, psychiatric nurse-specialist, and psychoanalyst in managing a suicidal patient were defined. Physician-assisted suicide and the dying patient's experience were discussed.

The important role of postvention, the things done after the event that help the individual who attempted suicide or help the suicide survivors, was emphasized near the conclusion of this chapter. The mourning experience for suicide survivors and the role of suicide survivor support groups were examined.

# RESOURCES

## Suicide and Life-Threatening Behavior on the Internet

American Association of Suicidology
www.suicidology.org

The American Foundation for Suicide Prevention
www.afsp.orf

Center for Elderly Suicide Prevention
www.gioa.org/program/cesp/cesp.html

Griefwork Center, Inc.
Offers professional educational programs on suicide postvention.
www.griefworkcenter.com

Grief Guidance, Inc.
Promoting intervention products and services for suicide survivors.
www.griefguidance.com

The National Hopeline Network
1-800-SUICIDE
Provides access to trained telephone counselors, 24 hours a day, 7 days a week.
www.1000deaths.com/hotline.html

SAVE — Suicide Awareness Voices of Education
The mission of SAVE is to educate about suicide prevention, eliminate stigma, and support those touched by suicide.
www.save.org

SPAN USA is dedicated to preventing suicide.
www.spanusa.org

Yellow Ribbon Suicide Prevention Program
An outreach program of the Light for Life Foundation International. Prevention training programs and crisis hotline.
www.yellowribbon.org

## CHAPTER 3
### Questions 25-38

25. The primary reason individuals complete an altruistic suicide is that they

   a. want to bring peace.

   b. feel as though they are not part of any group.

   c. believe they have no future.

   d. do not see any solution to their problems in a crisis situation.

26. The primary reason individuals complete an egotistic suicide is that they

   a. want to bring peace.

   b. feel as though they are not part of any group.

   c. believe they have no future.

   d. do not see any solution to their problems in a crisis situation.

27. The primary reason individuals complete a fatalistic suicide is that they

   a. want to bring peace.

   b. feel as though they are not part of any group.

   c. believe they have no future.

   d. do not see any solution to their problems in a crisis situation.

28. The primary reason individuals complete an anomic suicide is that they

   a. want to bring peace.

   b. feel as though they are not part of any group.

   c. believe they have no future.

   d. do not see any solution to their problems in a crisis situation.

29. In the United States, the highest suicide rate occurs in

   a. children under the age of 12.

   b. adolescents.

   c. adults (35 to 45).

   d. elderly (65+ years).

30. The type of suicide differentiated by less warning signs, more lethal means of ending life, and greater incidence of depression and physical illness is

   a. child.

   b. adolescent.

   c. adult.

   d. geriatric.

31. Suicidality patterns among lesbian, gay, and bisexual youths aged 14 to 21 years include greater incidence

    a. after they became aware of their sexual feelings and before they told their parents.

    b. after they became aware of their sexual feelings and after they told their parents.

    c. before they became aware of their sexual feelings and before they told their parents.

    d. before they became aware of their sexual feelings and after they told their parents.

32. Three physical illnesses associated with increased risk of suicide are

    a. AIDS, cancer of the brain, and multiple sclerosis.

    b. cancer of the liver, cancer of the lung, and cancer of the brain.

    c. cancer of the brain, multiple sclerosis, and cancer of the heart.

    d. AIDS, multiple sclerosis, and prostate cancer.

33. In 2001, the eleventh ranking cause of death in the United States is

    a. homicide.

    b. AIDS.

    c. suicide.

    d. car crashes.

34. The very concept of suicide intervention implies

    a. feeling anxious or unprepared when working with suicidal patients due to the level of training and experience.

    b. professional's attitudes toward suicide, their own history of suicidality, and death acceptance.

    c. an involvement in someone's intent to die, with that involvement averting the suicide.

    d. defining the problem, gathering information about the characteristics of the suicidal person, incidents and events that precipitated a suicidal act, and support received.

35. An active form of mercy killing is

    a. discussed assisted suicide.

    b. euthanasia.

    c. encouraged assisted suicide.

    d. accepted assisted suicide.

36. The term for when a clearly competent patient makes a voluntary request to a physician to administer a lethal dose of medication to end the patient's life is

    a. discussed assisted suicide.

    b. encouraged voluntary suicide.

    c. assisted voluntary suicide.

    d. voluntary active euthanasia.

37. The type of suicide that occurs when the physician discusses alternatives and encourages the individual to look at all of his or her options

    a. discussed assisted suicide.

    b. euthanasia.

    c. encouraged assisted suicide.

    d. accepted assisted suicide.

38. Those things done following a suicidal act that serve to mollify the after-effects in a person who has attempted suicide or to deal with the adverse effects on suicide survivors are called

    a. prevention.

    b. mass media reporting.

    c. imitation.

    d. postvention.

# CHAPTER 4

# CARING FOR THE DYING

## CHAPTER OBJECTIVE

After completing this chapter, the reader will be able to describe ways individuals cope with life-threatening illness and dying. This chapter focuses on how to provide support to those who are dying and explores the issues facing the family of the dying patient.

## LEARNING OBJECTIVES

After studying this chapter, the reader will be able to

1. differentiate between stage-based and task-based models for coping with dying.

2. differentiate between four types of death awareness contexts for dying patients and caregivers.

3. identify various health care systems' approach to dying.

## COPING WITH DYING

Kessler (1998) suggests ways to help the dying. Allowing the dying to be heard is one of the greatest gifts that we can offer. Medical professionals are taught that listening is a way of gathering information and assessing a patient's physical and psychological condition. Even more, listening itself is a powerful way of giving comfort. Loved ones and friends often arrive at the hospital in a panic,

afraid to see someone who is facing death. Not knowing what to say, they often turn to the nurse or doctor and ask: "What do we do? What do we say?" The answer is always to listen, just listen. Listen to them complain. Listen to them cry. Listen to them laugh. Listen to them reminisce. Listen to them talk about the weather or talk about death. Just listen (p. 21).

In her groundbreaking work, *On Death and Dying*, Kubler-Ross (1969) outlined the emotional stages the dying patient goes through. Not every dying person experiences each stage, nor do they occur in any particular order. In her model, the terminally ill recognize impending death as it proceeds through five stages of dying: denial, anger, bargaining, depression, and acceptance.

**Stage 1.** The initial response is *denial and isolation.* Denial acts as a buffer. Unable to take in the information, patients may seek out physicians for second opinions. Denial is a coping strategy, and some patients never move out of denial. A nurse should not attempt to move a patient from denial to acceptance.

**Stage 2.** Anger at anyone who is healthy is the second stage, which replaces denial. The patient may be angry at their quality of care. Allowing the patient to vent will help him or her deal with the anger. The patient may ask, "Why me?" There are no answers to this question. However, allowing the patient to ask this question will give the person the opportunity to feel rage and have an outlet for anger.

**Stage 3.** According to Kubler-Ross, the terminally ill also experience bargaining. They want to postpone the inevitable and attempt to enter into an agreement with God for more time. They may bargain to live until a goal is reached.

- A terminally ill patient bargains with God to attend her granddaughter's wedding.

- A dying mother tells her son that she would donate her body to science if only she could have more time.

**Stage 4.** Depression is the next stage. At this point, patients realize they are dying and feel sad about leaving all that is significant behind. They need reassurance, and the nurse can offer the gift of presence rather than false cheerfulness.

**Stage 5.** Eventually, the person comes to terms with dying, mourns the loss of self, others, and possessions, and reaches a kind of acceptance. Hope is not abandoned, as the person may still hope for a miracle.

Nurses are effective helpers if they look at the stages as a means for understanding where a person is in their coping process. Though these stages have been outlined, nurses should not feel obligated to manipulate and move those who are terminally ill through the stages. As the dying patient moves back and forth through all the stages, the nurse can focus on the stages as guideposts to recognize where someone is at a particular point in time. The stages do not appear in a fixed sequence. In fact, acceptance may never be achieved.

> **_Personal Insight_**
> *If your physician told you that you were terminally ill, what would you do with the time you had left?*

Another stage model of dying comes from a Buddhist perspective. According to Buddhism, there are eight stages to the dying process. For many

centuries, Buddhists have believed that as individuals go through each of the stages, changes occur bringing them closer to death.

Through the stages, the eyesight fades, the body becomes weak, the hearing dissolves, the body becomes numb, and the need to eat diminishes, until the person finally enters an unconscious state. Though there are eight stages in the dying process, Buddhists do not look at the last stage, death, as the end of a person's existence. In Stage 8, the person journeys into a new spiritual dimension.

The terminally ill may go through stages or have certain tasks to do before they die. A major task is to complete unfinished business (Kalish, 1985). Some of the ways terminally ill individuals can complete unfinished business is to make their spouse aware of the location of insurance documents and important papers, place a call to everyone in their address book, make up with a friend they have not seen in years, and tell special people in their life that they love them. Other tasks Kalish mentions include "dealing with medical care needs, allocating time and energy resources, arranging for what happens after death, coping with losses, and encountering the mysteries of death itself"(p. 153).

By addressing unfinished business, whether practical or emotional, the dying individual feels in control. Leichtentritt and Rettig (2000) note,

> "Two of the most important tasks that ought to be addressed while assisting a person to die are allowing an individual the opportunity to gain control over future events by specifying the manners in which s/he wished these rituals to be performed, and promising a dying person that s/he will be remembered and will live on through those left behind (p. 244).

Nurses play critical roles in addressing these two tasks.

Doka (1995-1996) describes how the tasks of coping change at various phases of the life-threatening illness. The *acute phase* is initiated by the diagnosis. The individual attempts to understand the disease, maximize health, develop coping strategies, explore the effect of the diagnosis, express feelings, and integrate the present reality into their sense of past and future. The *chronic phase* involves managing the symptoms and side effects while carrying out health regimes, normalizing life, and maximizing social support, at the same time as expressing feelings and finding meaning in the suffering. In the *terminal phase*, the individual copes with dying by managing the pain, symptoms, health procedures, and institutional stress. The dying prepare for death by saying goodbye and finding meaning in life and death. Some individuals have two other phases. The prediagnostic phase is when the individual suspects an illness and seeks out medical attention. The recovery phase is when the disease has been cured or is in remission.

Rando (1984) points out that during these phases, the terminally ill patient emotionally reacts to the situation and experiences certain feelings.

- Anxiety
- Fear of the unknown
- Fear of loneliness
- Fear of loss of family and friends
- Fear of loss of self-control
- Fear of loss of body parts and disability
- Fear of suffering and pain
- Fear of loss of identify
- Fear of sorrow
- Fears of mutilation, decomposition, and premature burial
- Depression
- Anger and hostility
- Guilt and shame

Byock (1996) notes that at the end of life those who are dying reach landmarks (see Table 4-1). At each landmark, the individual has taskwork to complete. These landmarks include completing one's

affairs, resolving relationships, having a sense of meaning in one's life and about one's life, experiencing love of self and others, acknowledging the finality of life and a sense of a new self, and letting go. By exploring landmarks and taskwork, the patient's quality of life is improved.

# DEATH AWARENESS

## Illness and Dying Trajectories

Does dying begin the moment the physician informs the patient of a terminal illness? If the patient does not believe the prognosis, is he or she still dying? Or does dying begin when the patient and physician both believe that nothing more can be done? When the physician believes that nothing more can be done to cure the patient, the physician will enter a dying trajectory. Glaser and Strauss (1968) have described the dying trajectory by setting up a graph with *time* along the horizontal axis and *nearness to death* along the vertical axis and then charting the patient's condition as time passes. The curve is the dying trajectory for that patient. The course of dying has duration and shape. It takes place over time, and it can move rapidly or slowly. It can be anticipated, with the patient and family members prepared, or it can happen suddenly. When the death happens suddenly, those in the patient's life are usually unprepared (Glaser & Strauss, 1968).

The time and nearness to death is different for each patient. The majority of individuals who have a life-threatening disease die in hospitals. Connor (1999) points out several general scenarios that can occur:

a. dying suddenly or after a short course of illness (MI, infectious disease, etc);

b. dying of a predictable downhill course of illness (cancer, ALS, etc.)

c. dying of a chronic illness with exacerbations, then converting to a more predictable course under palliative management; and

4. continuing with chronic illness, and intermit-

## TABLE 4-1: A WORKING SET OF DEVELOPMENTAL LANDMARKS AND TASKWORK FOR THE END OF LIFE

| Landmarks | Taskwork |
| --- | --- |
| Sense of completion with worldly affairs | Transfer of fiscal, legal and formal social responsibilities |
| Sense of completion in relationships with community | Closure of multiple social relationships (employment, commerce, organizational, congregational). Components include: expressions of regret, expressions of forgiveness, acceptance of gratitude and appreciation. Leavetaking; the saying of goodbye. |
| Sense of meaning about ones' individual life | Life review. The telling of one's stories. Transmission of knowledge and wisdom. |
| Experienced love of self | Self-acknowledgment. Self-forgiveness. |
| Experienced love of others | Acceptance of worthiness. |
| Sense of completion in relationships with family and friends | Reconciliation, fullness of communication and closure in each of one's important relationships. Component tasks include: expressions of regret, expressions of forgiveness and acceptance, expressions of gratitude and appreciation, acceptance of gratitude and appreciation, expressions of affection. Leave-taking; the saying of goodbye. |
| Acceptance of the finality of life — of one's existence as an individual | Acknowledgment of the totality of personal loss represented by one's dying and experience of personal pain of existential loss. Expression of the depth of personal tragedy that dying represents. Decathexis (emotional withdrawal) from worldly affairs and cathexis (emotional connection) with an enduring construct. Acceptance of dependency. |
| Sense of a new self (personhood) beyond personal loss | Developing self-awareness in the present. |
| Sense of meaning about life in general | Achieving a sense of awe. Recognition of a transcendent realm. Developing/achieving a sense of comfort with chaos. |
| Surrender to the transcendent, to the unknown—"letting go" | In pursuit of this landmark, the doer and taskwork are one. Here, little remains of the ego except the volition to surrender. |

*Source:* Byock I., (May 1996) The nature of suffering and the nature of opportunity at the end of life. *Clinics in Geriatric Medicine, 12*(2), pp. 237-251.

tent exacerbations until a final, difficult-to-predict demise.

## Awareness Contexts

*When a patient said to me, "I'm so glad you're my nurse today—because I wanted you to be the one with me on the day I die." She died at the end of my shift that day.*
— Larson, 1993

As the health professional shares information with the patient and or family member, each person becomes aware of the patient's condition. The awareness is based on information and how that information is perceived by the others. In their book, *Awareness of Dying*, Glaser and Strauss (1965) discuss four types of awareness contexts. In *closed awareness,* the patient does not know he or she is dying, but everyone else is aware. Often it is a family member who keeps the news from the patient. In *suspected awareness*, the patient suspects what others know and attempts to find out more information about his or her prognosis. Patients become suspicious as they become increasingly ill. They may simply want to know how sick they really are and not be told that they are dying. In *mutual pretense*, the patient, the family, and the staff pretend they do not know of the prognosis. In *open awareness*, the patient is aware of impending death, both preparing for it and discussing it.

Mak (2001) conducted a study of 33 Chinese hospice patients and found that all the patients in the study except one were aware that they were dying. Only one patient with cancer of the lung was kept in closed awareness. None of the patients pretended not to know they were dying. When individuals deny that they are dying or family members deny that their loved one is dying, it is a way of coping with the news. Weisman (1972) has proposed three degrees of denial:

1. denial of facts,

2. denial of implications, and

3. denial of extinction.

Weisman (1972) notes that in denying facts, a patient will be aware that, for example, the physician may be scheduling the patient for an operation for cancer, but the individual believes it is to remove a benign tumor. In denying the implications, the individual acknowledges the disease but not that he or she will die from it. Patients in denial of extinction may accept the diagnosis but still talk as though they were going to survive it.

Kalish (1985) refers to the process of dying in three ways:

1. as it is perceived by the person who is dying,

2. as it is perceived by other concerned persons, and

3. as it would be perceived by some objective qualified person who was privy to all knowable information

(p. 26).

## Addressing End-of-Life Concerns

What do the terminally ill want to know about their condition? Do they want to be told they are dying, and, if so, do they want to be told alone or with their families present? Would they prefer their physician inform their family members? Regardless of the approach, the language must be clear. Street and Kissane (1999-2000) note, "The words which surround a prognosis of a person with a progressive illness carry messages of finality and loss of hope; words such as incurable, no more active treatment, transfer to hospice, and terminal care" (p. 241). There is a conflict today between discussing end of life issues openly and attempting to spare individuals the pain of knowing they are dying. Kessler (1998) points out ways that health care professionals can discuss the patient's terminal disease by speaking in the positive.

- We can provide aggressive comfort treatment.

- We can set up a pain management program and reassess it constantly.

- We can allow open visiting.

- We can let you bring your pet.

- We can let you have pizza.

- We can improve the quality of the time you have remaining, making your last days or months as pleasant as possible.

- We can let you participate in the ending phase of your life.

- We can address your suffering and pain.

- And when the time comes, we can manage your dying, just as you want it (p. 55).

The stigma of death isolates those who are dying from their family and friends. Society pulls away from the dying at a time when they are most needed. Levetown, Hayslip, and Peel (1999-2000) note,

Physician reluctance to discuss end-of-life issues with patients may be caused by unsubstantiated fears of damaging their hope; by a perception that the physician's role is only to heal and reserve life; and by the feeling that such discussions should only occur in the context of an intimate relationship with the patient and family, relationships which are increasingly uncommon in modern medical practice (p. 325).

Nurses are an excellent resource to provide support and comfort to patients as their terminal illness is discussed. Patients generally would rather have a partial disclosure of the fact that they are terminally ill rather than non-disclosure, and they also prefer to be told of their prognosis in the presence of a loved one (Marwit & Datson, 2002). Patients remember every detail of the disclosure, from the tone of the medical practitioner, the date, the time, and the location to what happened after they were told (Mak, 2001).

Smith (2000) addressed end-of-life concerns and found that patients need to talk about death and dying. One question explored in the study was: "What do you think happens when a person dies?" Follow up questions were:

(a) how much participants think about their own death;

(b) what formal preparations they have made for dying and death (e.g. funeral, living will, power of attorney);

(c) where or from whom participants think they amassed their own ideas about dying and death;

(d) to whom they have spoken about dying;

(e) what kinds of information would be most important in making health care decisions at the end of life (e.g. cost of treatment, pain, opinion of significant others);

(f) a discussion of the deaths of persons close to the participant (especially parents) and the impact of these experiences on the participant; and

(g) how the participant would ideally like to die (p. 183).

Options to ease suffering in the terminally ill include therapeutic touch, which helps the terminally ill by promoting relationships and pain reduction. Music therapy can also be utilized in end-of-life care. Curtis' study of 17 terminally ill patients (O'Callaghan, 1996) reported that the music was effective in improving reduction of pain, physical comfort, relaxation, and contentment scores. Other studies have found similar results when the terminally ill listen to taped music. Lane (1992) reported that listening to music can benefit patients while they are undergoing painful procedures.

Incorporating massage therapy and the use of touch along with any pain medication will benefit the patient. Family members can be educated as to the importance of touch, as they may be hesitant to touch, afraid of causing additional pain to their dying loved one. Depending upon the response of the terminally ill, that touch may be exactly what is needed. Zuberbueler (1996) explains that massage reduces pain and slows the skin breakdown. A blending of certain oils and gentle massage is soothing and healing. According to Ellis, Hill, and Campbell (1995), when the caregiver or family member touches the patient, there is continued dialogue, and the family bond is strengthened during this difficult time.

With the concurrent use of pain medication, physicians can treat physical and emotional suffering with biofeedback, relaxation techniques, and transcutaneous electrical nerve stimulation (TENS). If relief cannot be obtained through pain medicine, treatments may include radiation therapy, nerve block, and surgery. It is of major significance to find the means to control the pain and deal with any underlying issues, including depression, in order to limit suicide ideation. It is particularly important to inform the patient that pain can ultimately be controlled because this information can significantly relieve the patient's anxiety. A direct solution to the problem of suicide ideation in the terminally ill is educating physicians about more effective pain management. This education can include incorporating family therapy and cognitive-behavioral methods along with complementary therapies in end-of-life care.

# PALLIATIVE CARE

During the past few years, there is an increased focus on palliative care, which enhances the patient's well-being in the last stages of life and helps them make peace with their situation (van der Kloot Meijburg, 2000). Many palliative care programs are developed for intense symptom management in the hospital. The purpose of palliative care is to reach the best quality of life, which includes pain management and psychological, social, and spiritual support for patients and their loved ones (Alaeddini, Julliard, Shah, Islam, & Mayor, 2000) The best possible quality of life for both the patient and family members is achieved when certain needs are met. Nurses should assess needs by devising a palliative care plan (see Table 4-2). These needs can

be as simple as having a private room available if the patient should want one and offering the family members a place to shower and sleep.

In December 1997, the Task Force on Palliative Care developed The Last Acts, a national coalition to improve care and caring near the end-of-life. The Last Acts Palliative Care Task Force believes that five core precepts should be acknowledged and incorporated into all end of life care (see Table 4-3). When providers acknowledge and respect patient goals, preferences and choices; exhibit comprehensive caring; utilize the strengths of interdisciplinary resources; acknowledge and address caregiver concerns; and build systems and mechanisms of support, the dying patient will receive the best possible quality of life near the end of their life.

Health professionals will offer aggressive comfort care during the end of life and alleviate suffering more effectively if they acquire related skills and competencies and are better educated in palliative care (Witt-Sherman, 1999). Palliative care benefits the professional, who receives great satisfaction in relieving the pain and suffering of their patients and improving their quality of their life. Palliative care includes symptom management of psychological as well as physical symptoms. Some of the physical symptoms include ascites, dyspnea, and fecal impaction (see Table 4-4). As nurses treat the physical symptoms, the patient and their family members must be educated about the medications, their benefits, and side effects. Symptom management can be a challenge to nurses as the patient's condition changes. Patient comfort is a priority.

Comfort care at the end of life includes teaching a patient proper wound care, safety measures, and diabetic care. If the patient is a diabetic, the nurse will teach the patient and caregiver how to check blood sugar, how to use a sliding scale, and how to inject insulin. Effective ways to use oral agents, the significance of foot care, signs and symptoms of infection, appropriate diabetic diet, and referral to a dietician should be discussed.

## TABLE 4-2: ASSESSMENTS NEEDED IN DEVISING A PALLIATIVE CARE PLAN

**Disease status and symptom assessment**

• What is the diagnosis and the prognosis?

• How is the disease likely to affect the patient?

• What other current physical or emotional problems (e.g., substance abuse) are relevant?

• What symptoms are present, and what symptoms are likely to emerge?

**Preferences and goals**

• Have patient and family preferences, beliefs, and goals been discussed?

• Has a surrogate decision maker been identified if the patient becomes unable to participate in decisions?

• Have appropriate documents been completed and preferences recorded in the patient's record?

**Emotional status and spiritual assessment**

• How does the patient feel about his or her situation?

• What are his or her hopes and fears?

• Should assistance from a pastor or other spiritual counselor be suggested or arranged?

• Has the patient been sufficiently assured that he or she will be cared for and will not be abandoned (assuming that reassurance can be truthfully offered)?

**Family assessment**

• How are family and closely involved others managing?

• How have they managed difficult situations in the past?

• How well do they understand the patient's condition and prospects?

• Do they need physical, emotional, or practical support?

• What special problems need attention (e.g., presence of young children in the home, other family illnesses, communication or cognitive problems, history of violence or substance abuse)?

**Functional status**

• What can the patient do for him or herself, and where is help required?

• What kind of assistance (e.g., removal of physical obstacles to bathroom access, total physical care) is needed and from what source?

**Therapy review and evaluation**

• What medications are being used and with what results? What potential drug interactions require monitoring?

• On the basis of patient status, should medications be continued, adjusted, or discontinued?

• What nonpharmacological therapies are being used or should be considered?

• What health care providers are involved in patient care? Is the level and mix appropriate?

• What are the benefits and burdens (for patient, family, and caregivers) of the therapies being provided, and what are the alternatives?

**Resource review and evaluation**

• What professional and nonprofessional personnel are available to support the patient and family?

• Are physical facilities in the home adequate (e.g., bathroom accessible)? How do transportation, economic, and other relevant resources match patient and family needs? What else can be done?

• Can resources be used more effectively or efficiently?

*Source*: Committee on Care at the End of Life. (1997). Chapter 3. In M.J. Field & C.K. Cassel (Eds.), *Approaching death: Improving care at the end of life* (p. 50-86). Washington, DC: National Academy of Sciences. Available online: http://www.nap.edu/readingroom/books/approaching/box3.4.html

If a patient is experiencing dysphagia and having difficulty swallowing, the nurse can refer the patient to a dietician. However, the nurse can also teach the patient and caregiver some guidelines for a pureed diet, soft diet, liquid diet, or reasons to avoid liquids. The nurse will assess nutritional states and may recommend small frequent meals and snacks as well as elevating the head of the bed during and for 1 hour after feeding.

Skin breakdown is another common problem. The patient and caregiver can be taught ways to manage the symptoms. Recommendations can

## TABLE 4-3: PRECEPTS OF PALLIATIVE CARE (1 OF 2)

### 1. Respecting Patient Goals, Preferences and Choices
**Palliative Care:**

- Is an approach to care that is foremost patient-centered and addresses patient needs within the context of family and community.

- Recognizes that the family constellation is defined by the patient and encourages family involvement in planning and providing care to the extent the patient desires.

- Identifies and honors the preferences of the patient and family through careful attention to their values, goals and priorities, as well as their cultural and spiritual perspectives.

- Assists patients in establishing goals of care by facilitating their understanding of their diagnosis and prognosis, clarifying priorities, promoting informed choices and providing an opportunity for negotiating a care plan with providers.

- Strives to meet patients' preferences about care settings, living situations and services, recognizing the uniqueness of these preferences and the barriers to accomplishing them.

- Encourages advance care planning, including advance directives, through ongoing dialogue among providers, patient and family.

- Recognizes the potential for conflicts among patients, family, providers and payors, and develops processes to work toward resolution.

### 2. Comprehensive Caring
**Palliative Care:**

- Appreciates that dying, while a normal process, is a critical period in the life of the patient and family, and responds aggressively to the associated human suffering while acknowledging the potential for personal growth.

- Places a high priority on physical comfort and functional capacity, including, but not limited to: expert management of pain and other symptoms, diagnosis and treatment of psychological distress and assistance in remaining as independent as possible or desired.

- Provides physical, psychological, social and spiritual support to help the patient and family adapt to the anticipated decline associated with advanced, progressive, incurable disease.

- Alleviates isolation through a commitment to non-abandonment, ongoing communication and sustaining relationships.

- Assists with issues of life review, life completion and life closure.

- Extends support beyond the lifespan of the patient to assist the family in their bereavement.

### 3. Utilizing the Strengths of Interdisciplinary Resources
**Palliative Care:**

- Requires an interdisciplinary approach drawing on the expertise of, among others, physicians, nurses, psychologist, pharmacists, pastoral caregivers, social workers, ancillary staff, volunteers and family members to address the multidimensional aspects of care.

- Includes a clearly identified, accessible and accountable individual or team responsible for coordinating care to assure that changing needs and goals are met and to facilitate communication and continuity of care.

- Incorporates the full array of inter-institutional and community resources (hospitals, home care, hospice, long-term care, adult day services) and promotes a seamless transition between institutions/settings and services.

- Requires knowledgeable, skilled and experienced clinicians, who are provided the opportunity for ongoing education, professional support and development.

*Source*: Last Acts, Task Force on Palliative Care. (1997). *Precepts of Palliative Care.* Available online: http://www.lastacts.org/docs/profprecepts.pdf

## TABLE 4-3: PRECEPTS OF PALLIATIVE CARE (2 OF 2)

**4. Acknowledging and Addressing Caregiver Concerns**
**Palliative Care:**

- Appreciates the substantial physical, emotional and economic demands placed on families caring for someone at home, as they attempt to fulfill caregiving responsibilities and meet their own personal needs.

- Provides concrete supportive services to caregivers such as respite, round-the-clock availability of expert advice and support by telephone, grief counseling, personal care assistance and referral to community resources.

- Anticipates that some family caregiving may be at high risk for fatigue, physical illness and emotional distress, and considers the special needs of these caregivers in planning and delivering services.

- Recognizes and addresses the economic costs of caregiving, including loss of income and non-reimbursable expenses.

**5. Building Systems and Mechanisms of Support**
**Palliative Care:**

- Requires an environment that supports innovation, research, education and dissemination of best practices and models of care.

- Needs an infrastructure that promotes the philosophy and practice of palliative care.

- Relies on the formulation of responsible policies and regulations by institutions and by state and federal governments.

- Promotes equitable and timely access to the full array of interdisciplinary services necessary to meet the multidimensional needs of patients and caregivers.

- Demands ongoing evaluation, including the development of research-based standards, guidelines and outcome measures.

- Assures that mechanisms are in place at all levels (e.g. systems, direct care services) to guarantee accountability in provision of care.

- Requires appropriate financing, including the development of new methods of reimbursement within the context of a changing health care financing system.

*Source*: Last Acts, Task Force on Palliative Care. (1997). *Precepts of Palliative Care.* Available online: http://www.lastacts.org/docs/profprecepts.pdf

include use of a moisturizer, putting a lubricant in the bath water, position changes on a regular schedule, using a water or eggcrate mattress, and wearing heel and elbow protectors.

As symptoms are managed, the nurse will explain that incontinence is a common symptom and describe care of the catheter and foley maintenance. If the patient is constipated or has diarrhea, the nurse will help the patient follow a bowel regimen. A nurse should assess bowel state, initiate dietary interventions, and teach the importance of increasing fluid, fruit, and fiber. Other common problems include hiccups, dry mouth, nausea, and altered breath patterns. For patients experiencing breathing difficulties, a nurse can teach the significance of pacing activities and breathing exercises. Due to breathing difficulties, the patient can grow weak. While assessing the level of weakness, a nurse can explain to the patient and caregiver the contributing causes of the weakness. A referral to an occupational therapist for an evaluation may benefit the patient. Providing assistive devices may also keep the patient safe.

In improving palliative care, nurses should stress medication compliance with patients and their caregivers for it is critically important to maintaining quality of life as the disease progresses. Alaeddini, Julliard, Shah, Islam, and Mayor (2000)

| **TABLE 4-4: PHYSICAL SYMPTOMS** |
|---|
| Ascites (hydroperitoneum): the accumulation of fluid in the peritoneal cavity, causing abdominal swelling. Causes include infections, heart failure, portal hypertension, cirrhosis, and various cancers (particularly of the ovary and liver). |
| Constipation: a condition in which bowel evacuations occur infrequently, or in which the feces are hard and small, or where passage of feces causes difficulty or pain. |
| Dyspnea: Labored or difficult breathing. Dyspnea can be due to obstruction to the flow of air into and out of the lungs, various diseases affecting the tissue of the lung, and heart disease. |
| Edema: Excessive accumulation of fluid in the body tissues; popularly known as dropsy. In generalized edema there may be a collection of fluid within the chest cavity (pleural effusions), abdomen (see ascites), or within the air spaces of the lung (pulmonary edema). It may result from heart or kidney failure, cirrhosis of the liver, acute nephritis, the nephritic syndrome, starvation, allergy, or drugs (e.g. phenylbutazone or cortisone derivatives). |
| Fatigue (asthenia): Mental or physical tiredness. |
| Fecal impaction: The end result of chronic constipation common in senile patients, often requires manual removal of the fecal bolus under an anesthetic. |
| Nausea: Feeling that one is about to vomit. Actual vomiting often occurs subsequently. |
| Pain: A localized or diffuse abnormal sensation ranging from mild discomfort to agony or distress, caused by stimulation of the functionally specific sensory nerve endings. |

*Source:* Bantam Books. (2000). *The Bantam Medical Dictionary,* (3rd rev. ed.). New York: Bantam.

summarize several physicians' recommendations for means of improving palliative care:

    a.   continuous involvement of the patient's primary care physician while the patient is receiving palliative care or is in a unit devoted to palliative care;

    b.   continuing education regarding pain management, especially for nurses and physicians;

    c.   educational courses for residents regarding the importance and nature of palliative care;

    d.   provision of pain management guidelines by hospital administration and legal services;

    e.   development of a means to encourage patients admitted to the hospital to initiate advance directives as soon as possible;

    f.   and close communication with health care professionals outside the palliative care setting regarding patients' needs during palliative care and terminal illness. (p. 81)

Palliative care includes encouraging terminally ill patients to participate in recreational activities. Ferszt, Massotti, Williams, and Miller (2000) looked at the benefit of an art program in an urban, 719-bed, academic medical and trauma setting. They polled two groups, with 7 patients in one group and 7 nurses in the other group. According to Ferszt et al., the majority of people in both groups benefited from the art program. It was noted that the separate art room allowed the patients to leave their own room and enjoy the relaxed, inviting environment. One patient said, "It gave me something to give to my children" (p. 194). Three nurses noted, "It gives you something to talk about besides the pain, their medication" (p. 196).

## Health Care Systems' Approach to Dying

Corr, Nabe, and Corr (2000) identified four programs of care for persons who are coping with dying.

1. Acute care: hospitals

2. Chronic care: long-term care facilities

3. Home care: home health care programs

4. Terminal care: hospice programs

## Acute Care: Hospitals

Hospitals are institutions that provide acute care, assessment, and diagnosis of illness, with cure-oriented treatment for conditions that can be treated (Corr, Nabe, and Corr, 2000). Lee (2003) notes, "The autonomy of technology has made possible rapid advances in medical knowledge in a system of healing that empower institutional approaches to health care" (p. 136). With these rapid advances, health care professionals attempt to meet the needs of the dying. Though they are efficient and trained, too often the health care professionals are overworked. This makes it difficult for them to give patients the time needed to address fears and concerns. Aiken (1994) describes the attitudes of medical personnel.

> Despite the availability of lifesaving equipment and medical expertise, a typical hospital or nursing home is not, from a psychosocial perspective, the best of all possible places in which to die. Busy physicians and nurses, who are preoccupied with administrative and technical duties, have little time to try to understand and deal with the emotional and social needs of dying patients. The hospital staff can be seen moving swiftly and efficiently in and out of intensive care rooms or terminal wards, checking their watches, administering medicines, and connecting, disconnecting, and tuning machines. If they do stop to chat with patients, it is usually only for brief moments before they are off to more pressing duties (p. 299).

## Chronic Care: Long Term Care Facilities

Another health care system is the nursing home, a long-term care facility that provides support to those who are chronically ill or dying. The nursing home becomes the residence, where people receive assistance with routine activities of daily living and can receive skilled nursing care if needed (Corr et al., 2000). Nurses in these facilities provide all types of care to meet the emotional, spiritual, and physical needs of patients and their families (Witt-Sherman, 1999). Those needs include breathing, diet, pain control, and security, the need to feeling safe and loved. Many of those who are chronically ill or dying reside in nursing homes and depend on their nurses to relieve them of their suffering. As family members visit their loved ones, the nurse can intervene by assisting family members with their emotional and spiritual needs. This can be done by educating them about what their loved one is currently experiencing, what the family may experience, and the dying process. By doing so, the family's fears and concerns can be alleviated as shown in the following example.

## Example

One morning, a visiting nurse was met at the door of her patient's home by John, the patient's husband. His wife's disease had progressed to the point where she had trouble breathing, was no longer eating or drinking fluids, and slept for most of the time. John appeared frightened and asked the nurse to wake his wife, Katie. She had not opened her eyes since the previous morning. After examining Katie, the nurse explained to John what happens to the body when death is near. As he touched Katie's skin, he asked about the discoloration of her face. The nurse reassured John that these symptoms were normal and that her pale face and bluish skin were normal colors when death is near. After mentioning that death was near, he asked the nurse how long his wife had to live. She told him that it could be a few hours or few days and that it was difficult to give him an exact moment. The nurse reassured him that his wife would be comfortable and not be in any pain. He told her that the issue that bothered him the most was her noisy breathing. The nurse explained Katie's breathing pattern. By reviewing with him that his wife's pain was being managed and her symptoms were normal, she helped him cope with his fears.

Nurses specializing in end-of-life care address the needs of their patients by talking with them and asking questions. These needs are not limited to symptom management and pain control. In fact, nurses can talk with their dying patients about their lives by exploring what the patient knows and providing support accordingly. The Institute of Medicine has made seven recommendations regarding the care of patients at the end of life approaching death. The testimony of Dr. Kathleen M. Foley to the Senate Committee on the Judiciary hearing stressed the need for health professionals to receive education regarding palliative care, patients receiving supportive care while pain is managed, and the available end-of-life options to patients and their families (see Table 4-5).

Woven through these important issues is the meaning of the patient's illness. A nurse can ask patients what is meaningful to them and what meaningful connections may have been lost or gained since becoming ill. Nurses can offer spiritual care by asking their patients about their source of strength, thus giving the patient permission to talk about what will happen to him or her as the disease progresses and what will happen after death. By listening and responding to the patient's spiritual needs, the nurse reinforces the meaning and purpose of the patient's life (see Table 4-6).

## Terminal Care: Hospice Programs

Saunders (1999) explains,

The word "hospice" as a welcome to travelers and the sick was first used in Rome in the late 4th century of the Common Era and taken to denote care for dying people in 1842 by Mme. Jeanne Garnier in Lyon, France. Down the centuries, innumerable unknown people have given exemplary care but the march today between "mind and heart" has opened up new possibilities of humanizing life a well as death (p. 6).

### Scope of Services

In 1974, Hospice Inc., the first United States hospice, opened its doors; it was later renamed Connecticut Hospice. There are 11,400 Home Health and Hospice Care agencies in the United States and 1.5 million Home Health and Hospice patients (National Center for Health Statistics, 2003a). Hospice is made up of an interdisciplinary team that includes a medical director, skilled nurses, spiritual and bereavement counselors, social workers, home health aides, and volunteers. The medical director oversees the patient's care and is instrumental in helping the entire team plan the patient's care plan. The nurse coordinates the patient's care and manages the symptoms. Hospice nurses are available outpatient or inpatient 24 hours a day and may visit regularly depending upon the condition of the patient.

Some hospices have a chaplain as a part of their interdisciplinary team to offer spiritual support to the patient and family members. The chaplains are also available to the staff as a resource to address their spiritual concerns as well. Other hospices hire a bereavement coordinator, and many restrict themselves to psychosocial counseling. Another part of the team includes the social worker, who looks at the family dynamics and seeks out community resources. The hospice social worker also assists the patient and family with any legal or insurance concerns. An integral part of the team is the hospice aide, who works closely with the hospice nurse and is often very much appreciated by the family.

### Example

Gina, a home health aide, cares for an 88-year-old hospice patient, Mrs. Clementi. Though she has only seen the patient three times, she senses that there is a possibility of high-risk bereavement for the patient's spouse. Mrs. Clementi lives with her husband, a 92-year-old retired handyman. All of their friends are deceased. She has hardly spoken with her husband since the physician informed her of her prognosis. Gina feels that he always seems angry. Gina contacted the hospice bereavement counselor, who recognized the high-risk bereavement signs, perceived a non-supporting social network, highly

## TABLE 4-5: INSTITUTE OF MEDICINE RECOMMENDATIONS ON THE CARE OF PATIENTS AT THE END OF LIFE APPROACHING DEATH

### RECOMMENDATION 1

- People with advanced, potentially fatal illnesses and those close to them should be able to expect and receive reliable, skillful, and supportive care.

### RECOMMENDATION 2

- Physicians, nurses, social workers, and other health professionals must commit themselves to improving care for dying patients and to using existing knowledge effectively to prevent and relieve pain and other symptoms.

### RECOMMENDATION 3

- Because many problems in care stem from system problems, policy-makers, consumer groups, and purchasers of health care should work with health care practitioners, organizations, and researchers to strengthen methods for measuring the quality of life and other outcomes of care for dying patients and those close to them; develop better tools and strategies for improving the quality of care and holding health care organizations accountable for care at the end-of-life; revise mechanisms for financing care so that they encourage rather than impede good end-of-life care and sustain rather than frustrate coordinated systems of excellent care; and reform drug prescription laws, burdensome regulations, and state medical board policies and practices that impede effective use of opioids to relieve pain and suffering.

### RECOMMENDATION 4

- Educators and other health professionals should initiate changes in undergraduate, graduate, and continuing education to ensure that practitioners have relevant attitudes, knowledge, and skills to care well for dying patients.

### RECOMMENDATION 5

- Palliative care should become, if not a medical specialty, at least a defined area of expertise, education and research.

### RECOMMENDATION 6

- The nation's research establishment should define and implement priorities for strengthening the knowledge base for end-of-life care.

### RECOMMENDATION 7

- A continuing public discussion is essential to develop a better understanding of the modern experience of dying, the options available to patients and families, and the obligations of communities to those approaching death

*Source*: Foley, K.H. (2000). Testimony of Dr. Kathleen M. Foley, Senate Committee on the Judiciary, Hearing entitles, "H.R. 2260, Pain Relief Promotion Act," April 25, 2000. Retrieved August 9, 2003, from http://www.senate.gov/~judiciary/oldsite/42520kf.htm

ambivalent relationship with the spouse, lower social class, and anger. Though the bereavement counselor will do an assessment after meeting with the patient and family, the aide is very much aware of the situation, and her assistance helps in the assessment of each patient. The aide was placing dishes into the dishwasher while Mr. Clementi sat at the table having a cup of coffee. He said, "I have never put a dish into the dishwasher. My wife has always done that

sort of thing. I wouldn't even know how to work it." She sensed that he was anxious in taking on roles his wife had done and knew that after her death, he would need to take on some of that responsibility. The aide said, "I can show you." He watched, listened, and then placed a dish in the dishwasher, put in the soap, and turned it on. Mr. Clementi thanked her several times. The aide used rehearsal, a tool that helps survivors practice new behaviors. She provid-

## TABLE 4-6: CARE FOR THE SPIRIT, THE ROLE OF SPIRITUALITY IN END-OF-LIFE CARE

Over time, western medicine has gradually separated the physical from the spiritual. But when medicine confront life-limiting illness and the promise of a cure dims, another approach is required. Confronting dying often brings with it questions such as, "Why me?" or "What will happen to me when life ends?" or "What has my life meant?" These are inherently issues of the spirit, not issues for biology or chemistry. Physicians and other health care providers increasingly recognize that good care of the dying is as much or more about these questions as it is about the relief of pain and symptoms.

- The word "religion" is often identified with adherence to a particular set of institutionalized belief systems and for some has a suggestion of the supernatural. The term "spirituality" is a more neutral term through which we acknowledge our common human need to find meaning in our lives and in our relationship to something beyond ourselves.

- **Spirituality**

  - is an expression of how a person related to a larger whole—that which an individual perceives as greater than him- or herself. The nature of this transcendent purpose can be expressed in different ways. For instance, it might be expressed through a specific religious tradition or, perhaps, through a regard for nature. For another person it might be expressed through connection to the human family itself or in some other way.

  - provides a source of meaning and understanding about the significance of being human. It addresses the question of "Why am I here?" An expression of spirituality can occur without any specific religious belief.

  - often contains habits, rituals, gestures and symbols that can help a person interpret and manage existence. Some of these may be acquired through or adapted from a specific religious tradition. Others may be ones that a person, family or community has developed.

- Religion, itself, plays an important part in the lives of Americans. A 2001 Gallup poll found 95% of those surveyed believed in God; 68% indicated they were members of a religious institution, and 44% had attended one in the past 7 days. 58% said that religion was "very important in life."

- Increasingly, medical schools are realizing that addressing spirituality can be an important and useful part of patient care. 61 medical schools now include some teaching about spirituality and medicine.

- In medical school courses on spirituality, students learn to work with many facets of spirituality and focus on the clinical integration of these themes into pregnancy, childbirth, chronic pain, psychiatric illness, addiction and dependency disorders, disability, and care of the dying.

- People want their doctors to ask them about spiritual concerns. A 1986 USA Today survey found that 63% of those surveyed believe it is good for doctors to talk to patients about spiritual beliefs.

- Research increasingly shows that spiritual practices have a positive effect on overall health and well being. By providing social support, such practices buffer stress and enhance coping.

*Source:* Last Acts, Task Force on Palliative Care. (2001). *Care for the spirit; the role of spirituality in end-of-life care.* Available online: http://www.lastacts.org/files/misc/careforspirit.pdf

ed him with an opportunity to practice using the dishwasher, which relieved some of his stress in taking on a new responsibility.

The support offered by aides includes taking care of the physical needs of the patient and light housekeeping duties. The assistance they offer the patient and family is very important. Their visits are usually longer than other members of the team and, more often than not, their presence gives the caregiver a much-needed break. Another essential part of the hospice team are volunteers, who are trained by the hospice. Lecture, group discussion, and reading material prepare the volunteer for their important role in providing inpatient or home care as well as bereavement support. A volunteer can go shopping, prepare meals, or babysit. For the most part, volunteers become friends with the patient and their caregivers.

The different educational backgrounds, talent, and experience create a hospice team that approaches the patient's care from various perspectives. A well-coordinated hospice team blends their roles in the patient's best interest. For example, when a family member discusses grief issues with the hospice nurse, immediate support is given to the family member. The bereavement or spiritual counselor is notified that additional assistance is warranted. Having knowledge of each other's disciplines creates a strong hospice group.

The hospice philosophy emphasizes palliative inpatient and home care. Though hospice services can be provided in the home, there is an increasing trend for hospice programs in hospitals, nursing homes, and free-standing facilities. The hospice philosophy stresses pain management and support to the psychological needs of the patient and their family. Emotional and spiritual support is provided as the patient's physical needs are met. For a year after the patient's death, bereavement support is made available to the family members.

Hospice philosophy is based on Cicely Saunders' aim to address the psychological need and pain of terminally ill patients. Her first visit to the United States in 1963 lasted 8 weeks, and during that time she met with doctors, psychiatrists, social workers, and chaplains to discuss care of the dying. In 1967 she opened St. Christopher's Hospice in England, with the aim of offering skilled compassionate care for the dying. Kastenbaum (1999) proposes that hospice makes a difference by providing the following help.

1. Reduction of pain and pain apprehension.
2. Reduction of cognitive clouding and confusion.
3. Improved communication.
4. Less sense of social isolation.
5. Preserved family bonds, not weakened.
6. Moderated depression and prevention of despair.
7. A flexible approach to terminal care that is responsive to the particular people and situation.
8. Reduction of the barriers to talking about dying and death.

Though most hospice care takes place in the patient's home, it can also be provided in a hospital, nursing home, or hospice facility. Haddad (1992) noted the advantages and disadvantages of interventions in the home. The advantages include:

a) the presence of family and familiar surroundings;

b) less danger of contracting infectious diseases;

c) less expense; and

d) greater opportunity for activity and participation in family life.

The disadvantages include:

e) increased family burden;

f) the invasion of family privacy;

g) the potential out-of-pocket costs for client and family; and

h) the absence of immediate professional care during an emergency.

Though hospice preserves family bonds, it is not easy for family members to take care of their dying loved ones. The responsibility of care still weighs heavily on the family member. Hospice teams are involved with the care of the patient. However, it is up to the family caregiver to provide most of the care, which can become emotionally and physically exhausting. Taking care of loved ones in the home can be a burden to families. Reinhard (2001) notes,

> Nurses in daily practice know that family caregivers are often asked to assume significant responsibilities without training in the

knowledge and skills required to fulfill these responsibilities. As the primary social group charged with the care of society's members, families are expected to be caregivers (p. 183).

The family caregivers may find peer comfort from volunteers, who provide family support and assistance with activities of daily living (Steinhauser, Maddox, Person, & Tulsky, 2000). Holistic care includes reading to patients or giving them reading material, visiting with their clergy, and writing (DeMong, 1997). Nolen-Hoeksema, Larson, and Bishop (2000) found that hospice family members reported hospice helpful and provided them with good information. However, those who reported more complaints about hospice were more likely to:

a.  be women,

b.  report the patient had needed a great deal of care,

c.  have a history of depression,

d.  have greater levels of distress before and after the patient's death, and

e.  be dissatisfied with the support they receive from family members and friends

> ### Personal Insight
> *How familiar are you with hospice? Would your recommend hospice?*

In 1982 the Medicare hospice benefit was created, which limits eligibility to those who have a medical prognosis of life expectancy of 6 months or less if the illness runs its normal course (Stuart, 1999). The certification of terminal illness is based on the physician's clinical judgment regarding the normal course of the illness. All Medicare-certified hospices in the same area reimburse at the same rates. These rates are determined by Medicare and not by the individual hospices.

*Advocacy*

The hospice team becomes an advocate for the patient. This is particularly true for the bereavement

coordinator. This bereavement professional serves as an advocate to promote attention to the grief and loss issues facing the patient, the family, the hospice staff, and the community at large. Bereavement coordinators can also offer support to the community, not limited to hospice patients and their families. Patients and family members can be referred to other organizations that support them, including local clergy. Bereavement coordinators are advocates as they support end-of-life research, refer patients and their families to support networks outside of hospice, help develop grief-related services to the community, and educate the public about hospice and the special needs of the terminally ill. The hospice bereavement professional can advocate for further research related to grief and loss issues.

*Assessment*

An essential component of hospice care is a careful assessment beginning with the presenting problem and moving through the individual's history. During this time, the health professional identifies what is paramount to the patient and family. The health professional addresses the physical changes that will take place. Even if they are competent in activities of daily living, this will help the patient understand and prepare for what will happen. By addressing these changes, the family can be realistic about the prognosis (Reese, 2000). The intake interview typically centers on introducing the patient and family member to hospice philosophy.

An ongoing assessment is made of the patient's physical, emotional, social, spiritual, economic, and intrapersonal needs. Current health and recent changes in health, feelings and history of grief, relationships and support systems, spiritual meanings, financial stability, and coping skills are assessed. Parker-Oliver (1999-2000) offers questions that health professionals can explore as they help their hospice patients and families cope:

> How is the family dealing with the fact that this person is dying? What are the goals of the family and the patient? How secure are

they with the dying process; How willing are they to let hospice assist in the process; and how committed are they to the hospice philosophy? (p. 503).

*Ethnicity and Culture*

As noted before, each culture has differences that hospice staff must respect. As the staff meets with patients and families, they will learn that each culture has different attitudes and beliefs about life and death. Hospice staff respect their patient's beliefs. For example, the followers of Hinduism fast on a regular basis, and a family member may fast on behalf of dying relative. They do this hoping to please a god who can bestow health. The followers of Islam may read from the Koran to their dying loved ones. This encourages those terminally ill to be patient with their suffering. The followers of Catholicism may request the sacrament of the sick. The hospice chaplain or bereavement coordinator can follow through on this request and contact a local priest. The priest anoints the dying with oil that has been blessed by a bishop. It is then massaged into the person's forehead.

Hospice staff must be mindful of ethnicity and cultural differences among their patients. A study comparing Caucasian and African-American reactions to death in Alzheimer's disease found more Caucasians died in facilities than African-Americans. Caucasian caregivers were more likely than African-American caregivers to withhold life-sustaining treatments, and Caucasians were more likely to be relieved after their loved one's death and to be less accepting of the death (Owen, Goode, & Haley, 2001). Knowing and respecting ethnicity and the cultural backgrounds of patients and their families will help hospice staff understand the choices they make regarding their care. Health professionals can meet the needs of those whose culture is different than their own, by collaborating with community agencies and educating themselves on issues related to culture.

*Bereavement Plan of Care*

After a patient is admitted to hospice, the patient and primary caregiver meet with the bereavement coordinator or spiritual counselor. As long as the patient is in hospice care, the bereavement coordinator will continue to assess the patient and the primary caregiver's need for grief support. Every hospice patient and their family will receive routine bereavement care unless they choose not to accept it.

All Medicare-certified hospices must provide bereavement support without charge to patients and families. Spiritual support is found as questions are explored through empathetic listening and life review. In a study by Thomson (2000), it was found that spiritual well-being raises a hospice patient's general quality of life and is a significant part of their life. However, hospice nurses and social workers are not trained to explore spiritual issues with their patient's families, caregivers, and patients themselves (Babler, 1997). By enhancing spiritual well-being, professionals will benefit the patient's physical well-being and overall quality of life (Thomson, 2000).

Hospice accepts patients of all ages, ethnicities, and mental capacities. When a person is dying, health care professionals provide support whether the patient is of normal intelligence or retarded. One hospice nurse for a 58-year-old mentally retarded patient wondered how she could prepare him for his death. She found that through his sharing of story, he was participating in a life review. She felt privileged to know him, help him prepare for his death, and learn from him about life (Helming, 2001).

Nurses work with dying patients at various time periods. In formulating a bereavement plan of care, the hospice spiritual counselor or bereavement counselor will provide the nurse with information and written materials on the dying process. These written materials can be offered to the family members of the hospice patients. The information in the pamphlets will describe to the nurses and family members what happens to the patient in the months, weeks, days, and hours leading up to their death. Nurses as well as the spiritual or bereavement counselors could review the material with the patient and family members.

Some of the information found in the material includes changes that may occur in the patient at 1-3 months prior to death, when the patient acknowledges their dying and begins to withdraw and communicate less with those around them, including neighbors, friends, and family. He or she may have no interest in watching TV or reading the paper and may be sleeping more than usual and taking naps throughout the day.

The information in the pamphlet will also include what happens 2 weeks prior to death, when a patient will most likely sleep for most of the day and night. The patient may be disoriented and often confused. Breathing changes can include puffing, blowing of the lips, and stopping of natural breathing only to start again. It is not unusual for those dying to speak with loved ones who are deceased. They may pick at the air, their pajamas or hospital gown, and their blanket. Physical changes include lowered blood pressure, changes in pulse, fluctuation in body temperature, and increased perspiration. The skin may appear blue or pale yellow.

The written material will also describe what occurs a few days before the patient's death. The patient may appear better, with their eyes open but not really seeing. He or she may ask for a meal or be alert, oriented, and ready for a conversation, when previously they did not want to talk. The patient may want to get out of bed and sit in the kitchen or living room to be with friends and family. They may appear restless, have irregular breathing, and be congested. The congestion at this time can be very loud. Hands and feet may appear purplish and blotchy.

### Bereavement Risk Assessment

After the patient dies, the nurse may attend the wake, funeral, or memorial service. The bereavement coordinator will visit the family to assess the bereavement needs and establish a bereavement plan of care. In helping the family cope with the death of their loved one, caregivers must look at risk factors for bereavement adjustment difficulty. The hospice bereavement coordinator or chaplain provides a risk assessment that relates the bereavement need to the service. Those with low risk for complicated bereavement have strong social supports and therefore telephone support may be all they need. There is some risk for adjustment if there are young children at home, lower social class, and unresolved previous losses. Low risk factors can include older age, their perception of social support, and sufficient financial resources (Walsh-Burke, 2000). High risk factors include a history of ineffective coping or a very high degree of dependence on the deceased. Those with high risk may need counseling or grief therapy to help them cope (Walsh-Burke, 2000). Those with some risk may want to participate in bereavement support groups or short-term individual bereavement counseling.

Nurses may see and hear things of which the bereavement and spiritual counselors are not aware. They can share this information with the hospice bereavement coordinator or chaplain, who will contact the patient's family to do a bereavement assessment. Some of the physical symptoms found during a bereavement assessment are shortness of breath, lack of energy, neck and shoulder pain, and rashes. Cognition can include hallucinations, preoccupation with the deceased, and confusion. Changes in sleep patterns, restlessness, visiting places where the deceased would have been, changes in appetite, and absentminded behavior are some behavioral issues. When doing a psychosocial emotional status assessment, it is not uncommon to note crying, sighing, anxiety, fatigue, anger, sadness, and denial.

Many hospice patients are elderly, and they leave behind loved ones who have experienced multiple losses in their life. They may experience personal death worries as they see their friends and loved ones dying around them. They may need to learn new skills as they adjust their roles. Although it is not uncommon to relocate, doing so should be well planned and not rushed.

Risks for complicated mourning are also assessed. The risks can range from intense grief to suppressing or postponing grief. By postponing grief, the bereaved avoid the pain of loss. The bereaved may not want to go home to an empty house, may become workaholics, and may make radical changes in their lifestyle. They may experience lowered self-esteem and isolate themselves from their friends and family. In the worst cases, they become violent or exhibit self-destructive behaviors.

Hospice provides ongoing support to the surviving family members after the death. This support creates a place for loved ones to feel a sense of emotional well-being as they take part in funeral planning and participation. Ragow-Obrien, Hayslip, and Guarnaccia (2000) found, "Individuals who used hospice also participated more in the various rituals surrounding the funeral . . . hospice users also perceived the funeral to be more meaningful than did traditional care users" (p. 302). Pastoral care in hospice is provided to patients and families in an attempt to find meaning in the illness, in life, and in death.

In smaller hospices, 20% of the nurses play a role in providing bereavement support, and 1% of the nurses provide bereavement support in large hospices (Foliart, Clausen, & Siljestrom, 2001). The spiritual counselor or bereavement coordinator plays a bigger role in larger hospices. However, every member of the hospice team should provide some type of bereavement support. Even though not all hospice patients and caregivers want a chaplain visit, hospice staff should be educated to discuss religious issues (Mickley, Pargament, Brant, & Hipp, 1998). By exploring the patient's religion, the hospice professional can explore their beliefs about life and the afterlife. By so doing, the patient can discuss not only their present situation but their future one as well. Foliart, Clausen, and Siljestrom (2001) found

that 98% of all hospices offered telephone support, 96% had scheduled mailings, 95% gave brochures about grief, 90% had pastoral visits, and 82% had volunteer visits. The results of this study underscore the value of providing support to the bereaved. A grieving individual feels supported when a professional calls them to see how they are coping. He or she appreciates receiving a mailing that invites them to a support group or candle lighting ceremony, as it gives the person an opportunity to share their pain of loss with others. When a brochure is received in the mail, the grieving person realizes that someone is thinking of them and they are not alone.

# SUMMARY

This chapter discussed the unique specialty area of caring for the dying. The chapter began with discussion of the stage-based and task-based models for coping with dying. The work of Kubler-Ross, who outlined the emotional stages the dying patient goes through, was noted. The Buddhist stage-based perspective on dying was also noted.

The chapter highlighted the phases in living with a life-threatening illness. How the tasks of coping change at various phases of the life-threatening illness were explored. At the end of life, those who are dying reach landmarks, and at each landmark the individual has taskwork to complete.

Focusing on illness and dying trajectories, several general scenarios that can occur were noted. Awareness contexts and how awareness is based on information and how that information is perceived by others were examined. Glaser and Strauss's four types of awareness contexts—*closed awareness, suspected awareness, mutual pretense,* and *open awareness*—were reviewed.

Within this chapter, the health care systems' approach to dying and the four programs of care for persons who are coping with dying were explored. The ways that hospitals, long-term care facilities, home health care programs, and hospice programs provide for those who are dying were discussed. As patients continue to die, there is an increase in focus on palliative care.

The chapter concluded by examining the hospice philosophy and the scope of services. Advocacy, assessment, community collaboration, ethnicity and culture, and the hospice bereavement plan of care were noted.

# RESOURCES

## Caring for the Dying on the Internet

Alzheimer's Disease and Related Disorders
    Association
    www.alz.org

American Academy of Hospice and Palliative
    Medicine
    www.aahpm.org

American Pain Society
    www.ampainsoc.org

Cancer Care, Inc.
    cancercare@aol.com
    www.cancercare.org

Hospice Foundation of America
    www.hospicefoundation.org

# EXAM QUESTIONS

## CHAPTER 4
### Questions 39-47

39. The five stages of dying in Kubler-Ross' model are

    a. denial, anger, sadness, depression, and acceptance.

    b. denial, anger, bargaining, depression, and acceptance.

    c. denial, anger, hope, sadness, and acceptance.

    d. denial, anger, hope, depression, and acceptance.

40. Two of the most important tasks that ought to be addressed while assisting a person to die are

    a. how the individual gains control over future events by specifying the manner in which he or she wished these rituals to be performed and promising the dying person that he or she will be remembered and will live on through those left behind.

    b. gaining control over present situation by being involved with all aspects of their health care and promising a dying person that he or she will not die in pain.

    c. offering the opportunity to meet with clergy and the funeral director.

    d. coping with various losses and making their spouse aware of the location of insurance documents.

41. The phase in which an individual copes with dying by managing the pain, symptoms, health procedures, and institutional stress is the

    a. acute phase.

    b. chronic phase.

    c. terminal phase.

    d. prediagnostic phase.

42. The curve on a graph of a terminally ill individual's dying trajectory shows the process

    a. occurring suddenly or after a short course of illness.

    b. taking place over time and moving fast or slow.

    c. related to time along the vertical axis and nearness to death along the horizontal axis.

    d. related to time along the horizontal axis and nearness to death along the vertical axis.

43. The type of awareness of a patient who does not know he or she is dying even though everyone else is aware is

    a. closed awareness.

    b. suspected awareness.

    c. mutual pretense.

    d. open awareness.

44. The awareness of a patient's impending death when the patient, the family, and the staff pretend they do not know of the prognosis is

    a. closed awareness.

    b. suspected awareness.

    c. mutual pretense.

    d. open awareness.

45. The type of care described as a means of reaching the best quality of life, which includes pain management and psychological, social, and spiritual support for terminally ill patients and their loved ones is called

    a. cumulative care.

    b. death and dying care.

    c. palliative care.

    d. compassionate care.

46. The type of institution where an individual lives, is helped with the routine activities of daily living, and is offered some level of assistance or skilled nursing care is called

    a. acute care: for example, hospitals.

    b. chronic care: for example, long-term care facilities.

    c. home care: for example, home health care programs.

    d. terminal care: for example, hospice programs.

47. The advantages of hospice providing interventions in the patient's home include

    a. the presence of family and familiar surroundings.

    b. more danger of contracting infectious diseases.

    c. less opportunity for activity and participation in family life.

    d. increased family burden.

# CHAPTER 5

# END-OF-LIFE DECISION-MAKING

## CHAPTER OBJECTIVE

After completing this chapter, the reader will be able to describe advance directives and issues facing individuals at the end of their life and their family members.

## LEARNING OBJECTIVES

After studying this chapter, the reader will be able to

1. describe the purpose of informed consent.

2. recognize the purpose of an advance directive.

## END-OF-LIFE DECISION-MAKING

### Informed Consent

Ethically and legally, patients have the right to be included in the decision-making process regarding their health care. Informed consent is a legal doctrine where the physician is required to inform patients about their condition and any risks involved in treatment. The informed consent form marks the fact that communication, a dialogue and process, between the practitioner and client has taken place. Throughout the dialogue and process of informed consent, the health professional should assess the patient's understanding of what is being said. It is not uncommon for patients to feel intimidated by health care professionals who ask them to sign a form regarding their health care.

During the informed consent process, the health care professional may make recommendations but also must discuss all possibilities in lay terms so the patient understands what is being asked. The competent patient is offered reasonable choices to the proposed intervention and, in making the decision, accepts or rejects the intervention. Though competence is a legal term, with the determination of a patient's competence sometimes made by a court of law, routine assessment is made by the patient's attending physician.

### Ethical Issues

In addressing the choices patients have regarding their end-of-life care, we must recognize the significance of ethical issues and the fundamental rights of patients. Rules and regulations are based on laws. There are individuals being kept alive in a coma or are in a persistent vegetative state. Ethically, does the health care professional need to know the patient's wishes to discontinue artificial means of life support? Who makes the decision to keep that patient alive? Ethics are systems of moral values that guide us in our conduct and treatment of individuals. Health professionals establish sets of moral standards known as a code of ethics. Ethics can be viewed simply as knowing and doing what is right. In doing what is right, legal issues must be acknowledged. One legal issue is withholding or withdrawing life-sustaining treatment (i.e. medication that could prolong the person's life, such as a ventilator or feeding tube).

## Advance Directives

A living will and a durable power of attorney for health care are two types of advance directives. The durable power of attorney allows the individual to name a representative to make health care decisions on their behalf. The living will, otherwise known as an instruction directive, is where an individual indicates the kinds of medical treatments they would accept or reject in different situations. Both are recognized under state law relating to the provision of health care when the individual is incapacitated. Each state regulates advance directives differently; many states' laws honor out-of-state advance directives as long as there is no conflict with that state's law. Upon admission to a healthcare agency, hospital, skilled nursing facility, or hospice program, patients should be made aware of how far the providers will go to comply with their wishes. Written policies should be in place that guarantee patients will be given written information on advance directives.

> *Personal Insight*
> *Are you comfortable asking a patient if they have an advance directive? Explore the reason for your feelings.*

Some physicians are uncomfortable talking about advance directives. Physicians sometimes want to oversee the process as a nurse or legal expert discuss advance directives with their patients (Alaeddini et al., 2000). Though chaplains, social workers, psychiatrists, and lawyers may talk with individuals about advance directives, physicians also should discuss this document with their patients. The document then becomes a part of their medical records. Home care and hospice nurses can also ask crucial questions and direct patients to the right resources (Norlander & McSteen, 2000). Nurses attempt to find out their patients' under-

standing of their illness, to understand if they perceive it as life-threatening or curable, and to determine whether there are any options regarding treatment. Taking a patient's past history of death experiences is an important part of understanding his or her present wants and needs. If the patient was ever with a dying family member or loved one, how that person died may directly affect their preferences for their own end-of-life care.

As the health professional attempts to find out the patient's wishes, identifying the patient's support systems is important. The patient's family can be included in the decision-making process as the patient decides what is in the best interest of themselves and their family. The patient can then decide whom to identify as their healthcare agent. Patients may choose where and to some degree how to die. However, note that advance care planning can take time. The questions and answers do not need to be decided in one visit. As patients become more comfortable in discussing their own wants, they also become more comfortable addressing these wishes with their physician. Individuals can always change their mind and either change or revoke their advance directive. Norlander and McSteen (2000) recommend the following open-ended questions to identify the patient's perspective on their illness.

- "It appears your condition is changing. What has the doctor told you?"

- "You've been hospitalized three times in the last 2 months. Tell me how this has been for you."

- "Have you talked with your family about your health?"

- "How are you coping with all of this?"

- "What is your understanding of your treatment options and your prognosis?"

- "Do you have any fears about your illness getting worse?"

(p. 538).

Professionals may initiate discussion with their patients regarding advance directives to determine their preferences, or patients may discuss their wishes on their own accord with family caregivers (Pickett, Barg, & Lynch, 2001) If the person is in a health care facility, in most states, the physician and facility are legally bound in an emergency to honor the decision of the patient or those who speak for them (e.g., a surrogate). Unfortunately, advance directives are often overlooked in an emergency, as there is no time in an emergency either to consult the advance directive or to determine a person's underlying medical condition.

Men and women, when faced with choices concerning the end of their life, generally have different preferences. As more men expressed a stronger preference for life-sustaining treatment than women, given their current health, more women expressed a greater desire to have a dignified death than men. Women may not want to live with diminished cognitive and social abilities and so they may choose not to have life-sustaining treatment (Bookwala et al., 2001). It is the right of every man and woman to make their own health care decisions at the end of life. This can be accomplished by filling out an advance directive, an oral or written instruction, about their own future medical treatment, in case they become unable to speak for themselves.

## Living Wills

A living will is a type of advance directive in which a person's wishes about medical care are written, in case the person is unable to communicate at the end of life. Each state may by law define when the living will goes into effect and may limit the treatments to which the living will applies. In order to make an advance directive, the individual must be at least 18 years old. A living will can also include the information that a person wants all possible medical treatment to prolong life.

*Personal Insight*
*Do you have a completed advance directive? If you do not have an advance directive, why not?*

## Do Not Resuscitate (DNR) Orders

A Do Not Resuscitate (DNR) order is an advance directive that is accepted by physicians and hospitals in every state. In the case where a patient's heart stops beating or the patient is unable to breathe, the DNR is a written request not to have cardiopulmonary resuscitation (CPR). A patient must fill out an advance directive form or inform their physician they do not want to be resuscitated. If the patient fills out the form, the physician puts a DNR order in the patient's medical records. The restrictions the patient places on use of CPR are based on certain anticipated physical conditions or quality of life issues.

*Personal Insight*
*What is most significant to you, the quality or the length of your life?*

Patients in extreme physical illness, such as whose cancer has spread or who find out they have Alzheimer's disease or whose kidneys are failing, may decide to choose DNR. However, some patients want everything done to stay alive, no matter what their condition. Patients need to be informed that if they choose DNR, other treatments will still be made available to them, such as treatment for pain, use of a ventilator, and transfusions. For those who are terminally ill, a DNR order is a valuable tool in avoiding needless invasive treatment.

The focus of an advance directive is on the individual's values and not only the medical intervention. The patient and their family members can complete a values exercise with their health care professional to clarify their expectations and fears in clinical circumstances (see Figure 5-1). Because the actual clinical circumstances rarely follow what is written in the directive, the physician has to interpret what the patient wanted in each scenario (see Figure 5-2). When a person fills out the advance directive, they cannot predict what will happen to them. Though a patient may indicate certain preferences,

## FIGURE 5-1: VALUES QUESTIONNAIRE

The following questions can help you think about your values as they relate to medical care decisions. You may use the questions to discuss your views with your health care agent and others, or you may write answers to the questions as a help to your agent and health care team. (If you fill out this worksheet and want it to be part of your DPA/HC, sign it in the presence of witnesses and attach it to your DPA/HC form.)

1. What do you value most about your life? (For example: living a long life, living an active life, enjoying the company of family and friends, etc.)

2. How do you feel about death and dying? (Do you fear death and dying? Have you experienced the loss of a loved one? Did that person's illness or medical treatment influence your thinking about death and dying?)

3. Do you believe life should always be preserved as long as possible?

4. If not, what kinds of mental or physical conditions would make you think that life-prolonging treatment should no longer be used? Being:
   - unaware of my life and surroundings;
   - unable to appreciate and continue the important relationships in my life;
   - unable to think well enough to make every-day decisions;
   - in severe pain or discomfort;
   - other (describe).

5. Could you imagine reasons for temporarily accepting medical treatment for the conditions you have described? What might they be?

6. How much pain and risk would you be willing to accept if your chances of recovery from an illness or injury were good (50-50 or better)?

7. What if your chances of recovery were poor (less than one in 10)?

8. Would your approach to accepting or rejecting care depend on how old you were at the time of treatment? Why?

9. Do you hold any religious or moral views about medicine or particular medical treatments? What are they?

10. Should financial considerations influence decisions about your medical care? Explain.

11. What other beliefs or values do you hold that should be considered by those making medical care decisions for you if you become unable to speak for yourself?

12. Most people have heard of difficult end-of-life situations involving family members or neighbors or people in the news. Have you had any reactions to these situations? If so, describe:

**Date** _____ **Signature** _____ **Date of Birth** _____

**Address** _____

**Witness** _____ **Witness** _____

*Source:* Vermont Ethics Network, 89 Main Street (City Center), Drawer 20, Montpelier, VT 05620-3601 (802)828-2909, www.vtethicsnetwork.org/worksheet1.htm

## FIGURE 5-2: MEDICAL SITUATIONS AND THEIR TREATMENT

This worksheet presents possible treatment plans for a variety of common medical situations. You may use these examples to discuss your views with your health care agent and others, or you may write down your choices as a help to your agent an health care team. (If you fill out this worksheet and want it to be part of your DPA/HC, sign it in the presence of witnesses and attach it to your DPA/HC form.)

**Possible Treatment Plans**

A.  I would want all possible efforts to preserve life as long as possible.

B.  I would want comfort care only, and would not want medical treatment, including tube-feeding, to prolong my life.

C.  I would want comfort care and tube-feeding but would not want other types of medical treatment to prolong my life.

D.  My agent should consider the possible benefits and burdens of disease-fighting treatment, and consent only to treatment that he or she believes is in my best interests, as we have discussed them. My agent may refuse any active treatment or may consent to a trial of treatment and then stop treatment if it is not beneficial.

**Possible Medical Situations**

1.  Suppose you have a fatal ("terminal") condition. You are unconscious and death is expected soon, with or without treatment. What treatment would you want? (Select from above, or write your own.)

2.  Suppose you are permanently unconscious from an accident or severe illness. There is no reasonable hope of recovering awareness, but life support could keep your body alive for years. (This is called "persistent vegetable state" or "permanent coma.") What treatment plan would you want? (Select from above or write your own.)

3.  Suppose you are in a state of very advanced loss of mental capability, due perhaps from stroke or Alzheimer's disease. You cannot recognize or communicate with those close to you, and can do almost nothing for yourself. You could survive in this state for some time with medical treatment. What treatment plan would you want? (Select from above, or write your own.)

4.  Suppose you are in a state of permanent but not total confusion, perhaps from stroke or Alzheimer's disease. You are legally "incompetent" and cannot recognize people and interact with them in a meaningful way, but you are up and around and people are taking care of you. You are not in distress and seem to be able to experience some satisfactions in daily life, such as eating or hearing music. Then you get an illness that might be fatal. What treatment plan would you want? (Select from above, or write your own.)

5.  Suppose you are frail, chronically ill and uncomfortable, with a limited range of activities available to you. Then you become unconscious, at least temporarily, due to an acute illness. The illness is likely to be fatal unless vigorously treated in a hospital but even intensive care offers only a small change of recovery to your former condition. It's much more likely that you will end up worse off than before, or will die in spite of all heroic measures. What treatment plan would you want? (Select from above, or write your own.)

6.  Suppose you unexpectedly suffer a serious injury or illness. You have less than a 5 percent chance of good recovery and, if you survive, will have serious brain damage. What treatment plan would you want? (Select from above, or write your own.)

7.  Use this space to describe any other medical situations you'd like to address:

*Source:* Vermont Ethics Network, 89 Main Street (City Center), Drawer 20, Montpelier, VT 05620-3601 (802)828-2909, www.vtethicsnetwork.org/worksheet1.htm

the reality is not always quite like what the person has checked off on their advance directive.

## Example

As a patient discusses DNR with her physician, she confidently says, "I never want to be put on a ventilator. A ventilator is never an option no matter what." However, the physician informs her that if she were able to come off the dependency of the machine in a few days or weeks, under those circumstances, would she still want a breathing machine. The patient says, "In that case, I would definitely want to be on a ventilator." If the physician did not explore various circumstances, he would not have understood the patient's true wishes and that she would want to pursue the short-term treatment option. When discussing DNR, make the distinction between long-term, short-term, or not doing anything at all in a particular scenario.

## Health Care Proxy

A medical power of attorney, also known as a health care proxy, is a document that allows the patient to appoint someone they trust to make decisions about their medical care if they are incapacitated. This trusted individual becomes their health care agent through creation of a durable power of attorney for health care. Though some of the clinical situations may be unclear, the patient gives the agent full authority to use their discretion. The authority is given based on the facts and what that person knows about the patient.

The durable power of attorney for healthcare authorizes the agent to speak for the patient when they become incapacitated, not only at the end of the patient's life. If the patient becomes mentally incapacitated, the health care proxy still remains in effect.

Norlander and McSteen (2000) note that asking a patient if they want to be resuscitated if their heart stops ignores "the larger context and history of the person's illness and life" (p 533.) Linda Norlander, Project Director for the Allina End of Life Project, helped develop an advance care planning discussion

model, *The Kitchen Table Discussion*, for health care professionals. The focus here is on the discussion that takes place between the health professional, the patient, and the family members. It begins with the patient's understanding of the illness; their personal death experiences, and their goals and values. This empowers them to communicate with their doctor. The discussion explores how the family is supporting the goals and values of the patient. This advance care planning discussion includes giving the patient and family more personal resources (Norlander & McSteen, 2000). As health care professionals, nurses may be called upon to assist terminally ill individuals and their families as they make their advance planning. By providing accurate and current information, nurses can address the patient's fears and the possible misconception that nothing will be done.

## Five Wishes

Five Wishes was created by the founder of Aging with Dignity, Jim Towey, with the assistance of physicians, nurses, lawyers, and experts in end-of-life care. Jim believed that an easy-to-understand health agent form was needed that would help the individual express how they would like to be treated if seriously ill and unable to speak for themselves. He created Five Wishes, a document that addresses the person's medical, personal, emotional and spiritual needs and encourages discussing wishes with family and physicians. The form, which is simple to use, reviews Five Wishes.

1. The person I want to make care decisions for me when I can't.

2. The kind of medical treatment I want or don't want.

3. How comfortable I want to be.

4. How I want people to treat me.

5. What I want my loved ones to know.

Organizations such as churches, synagogues, hospices, hospitals, medical, and legal offices, and social service agencies are distributing this document in 35 states and the District of Columbia. Five Wishes speaks in plain language and is easily understood by those who are not lawyers or physicians. Health professionals can advise their patients to make an advance directive, like Five Wishes, before they become seriously ill. In case of a health crisis where they cannot speak, their doctor and family will then know exactly what their wishes are, as the form will speak for them.

If you are asked to help someone fill out Five Wishes, first examine the document with them. In picking the right caring individual to be their health care agent, have them choose someone who knows them very well. Whomever they choose, this person must be able to stand up for them so that their wishes are followed. As they fill it out, the nurse should help them follow the directions and make sure that both the patient and the agent sign it. Remind your patient to discuss the Five Wishes with their family members and physicians and to make copies for them. Inform patients that they can change their minds at any time.

## The Patient Self-Determination Act

The Patient Self-Determination Act is a federal law that was passed by Congress in 1990. The act requires a health agency, hospital, skilled nursing facility, or hospice program to inform all adult patients about their rights to accept or refuse treatment and the right to execute an advance directive. Hosay (2003) notes, "Refusal to comply with a directive, for any reason, pits the rights of a patient to have his or her wishes honored against the rights of a provider to refuse care for reasons of conscience" (p. 152). If the advance directive goes against the policies of the facility (e.g., physician-assisted euthanasia), the patient should be informed.

## Tissue, Organ, and Body Donation

As of October 11, 2003, there are 82,896 people on waiting lists for organ donation (United Network for Organ Sharing). Donation is the act of giving one's organs or tissue to someone else. It is illegal to sell human organs or tissues. The United States Department of Health and Human Services maintains that transplantation saves lives. Approximately 63 people each day receive organ transplants because an individual said "yes" to organ and tissue donation on a donor card and/or on a driver's license.

Donors should carry their donor card with them to make their wishes known immediately. It is also important to discuss their decision with their family. The nurse may have to provide grief support to family members as they decide whether or not to donate their loved one's organs. Even in cases where the individual has requested that the organs be donated, organ retrieval is not allowed without the family's consent, as shown in the following example.

## Example

Sally and Frank arrived at the hospital and were told that their 21-year-old daughter, Anne, was in critical condition following a car accident. Anne was being kept alive by a ventilator and was considered brain dead. The nurse prepared them for what they would see and explained the reasons for the machines, tubes, and equipment. The hospital had a system in place to discuss organ donation with family members. The hospital staff introduced the subject of organ and tissue donation in a caring and compassionate manner. Though Anne had checked the back of her driver's license to indicate she was a donor, her father was against organ donation. He said, "I won't have them cut her up. She won't even be able to have an open casket." Sensing his fear and need of guidance, the hospital staff addressed his concerns and discussed that the appearance of Anne's body would not be changed. He was assured that his daughter's body would be treated with respect and dignity. The casket could remain open and no one would know that she was an organ donor unless they were told. Though Sally and Frank did not believe in organ donation and felt torn between their own beliefs and their daughter's, they respected their daughter's wishes. They allowed the dona-

## TABLE 5-3: NATIONAL DONATE LIFE MONTH

Advances in medical research and technology are helping our citizens to live longer and better lives. An important aspect of these improvements is transplant technology. Today, up to 50 lives can be saved or enhanced by just one organ and tissue donor. During National Donate Life Month, we honor living and deceased donors and their families across our Nation who have renewed the lives of others, and we call upon more Americans to follow their example.

Through our Nation's organ and tissue donor programs, thousands of Americans have given the gift of life. In 2002, 24,851 organ transplants and 32,744 corneal transplants were performed in the United States. In addition, the National Bone Marrow Donor Registry facilitated an average of 173 transplants each month. These donors' spirit of giving reflects the compassion of our great Nation.

Unfortunately, the current rate of donation is inadequate to meet the growing needs of our fellow Americans. Nearly 81,000 of our citizens are on the national organ transplant waiting list. Each day, an average of 68 of these individuals receive an organ transplant, yet another 17 on the waiting list die. As a Nation, we must strive to meet the needs of all Americans awaiting such donations. Through the "Gift of Life Donation Initiative," my Administration is working to educate our Nation about the importance of becoming a donor. During National Donate Life Month, more than 6,000 partners, including Federal agencies, State governments, private industries, unions, fraternal organizations, and associations have committed to promoting organ and tissue donation awareness. As a result, millions of Americans will learn about the many ways they can help those in need and save lives

NOW, THEREFORE, I, GEORGE W. BUSH, President of the United States of America, by virtue of the authority vested in me by the Constitution and laws of the United States, do hereby proclaim April 2003 as National Donate Life Month. I call upon our citizens to sign an organ and tissue donor card and to be screened for bone marrow donation. I also urge healthcare professionals, volunteers, educators, government agencies, and private organizations to help raise awareness of the important need for organ and tissue donors in communities throughout our Nation.

IN WITNESS WHEREOF, I have hereunto set my hand this first day of April, in the year of our Lord two thousand three, and of the Independence of the United States of America the two hundred and twenty-seventh.

GEORGE W. BUSH

*Source:* Bush, G. (2003). http://www.whitehouse.gov/news/releases/2003/04/20030402.html

tion to take place, and Frank signed the consent form. Though they were not interested in keeping track of Anne's gifts, the organ procurement coordinator told them that this was an option, as well as being able to communicate with the recipient through anonymous letters forwarded by the coordinator. The hospital staff recommended that Sally and Frank attend a donor family support group, a place to tell their story and discuss Anne's life. They attended several meetings, where they asked questions and shared their feelings with other grieving families.

Anyone over the age of 18 can agree to be a donor; those under 18 must have their parent's consent. When someone dies who has not filled out a donor card, their next of kin can donate their organs and tissues at the time of death. Newborns as well as senior citizens can become donors. After the death of someone under the age of 18, parents or legal guardians make the decision about donation. This is called non-living donation. At the time of death, medical suitability for donation is determined. Recipients are matched to organs based on blood and tissue typing, medical urgency, time on waiting list, and geographical location. There is no cost to the donor family; all costs are paid by the recipient, usually through insurance, Medicare, or Medicaid (DHHS—First Gov).

There is almost always some brief time lapse between the actual trauma and the declaration of brain death. During this period, the patient is supported with a ventilator—initially in an attempt to save the life, eventually to maintain the organs for transplantation. Without this forewarning, there could be no organ donation. Only patients who experience total cessation of brain function, including that of the brain stem, and who are being maintained on ventilators can provide viable organs for transplantation (Holtkamp, 2000).

In some circumstances, such as advanced age or medical condition, a patient may not be eligible for donation. If a family member wants to donate their loved one's organs or tissues and are told they cannot do so, the family member may feel disappointed and saddened. Being able to renew the lives of others through donation can bring comfort to survivors and victims. When the option of donation is not available to family members, it can be upsetting.

> *Personal Insight*
> *Are you a donor? What factors influenced your decision in being or not being a donor?*

On April 2, 2003, the Office of The Press Secretary for the President of the United States, sent out a press release recognizing April, 2003 as National Donate Life Month (see Figure 5-3).

# SUMMARY

This chapter began with a discussion of informed consent and the patient's right to be included in the decision-making process regarding his or her health care. Ethical issues and the fundamental rights of patients were noted. Advance directives, the oral or written instruction about a person's future medical treatment in the event they become unable to speak or make decisions, were discussed. Living wills, Do Not Resuscitate (DNR) orders, Five Wishes documents, durable powers of attorney for health care, and health care proxies were presented. The Patient Self-Determination Act was reviewed. Finally, this chapter ended with a discussion of tissue, organ, and body donation.

# RESOURCES

## End-of-Life Decision-Making on the Internet

Americans for Better Care of the Dying
    http://www.abcd-caring.org/

Coalition on Donation
    http://www.shareyourlife.org

Compassion in Dying Federation
    http://www.compassionindying.org/index.php

Last Acts
    www.lastacts.org

National Hospice and Palliative Care Organization
    http://www.nhpco.org

Organ and Tissue Donation/Transplantation —
    Donate Life
    http://www.organdonor.gov

Vermont Ethics Network
    http://www.vtethicsnetwork.org

United Network for Organ Sharing (UNOS)
    http://www.unos.org

# EXAM QUESTIONS

## CHAPTER 5
### Questions 48-54

48. A legal doctrine where the physician involves the patient, informs them of their condition, and discusses any risks involved in treatment is

    a. DNR.
    b. the Patient Self-Determination Act.
    c. informed consent.
    d. ethics.

49. Systems of moral values that guide us in our behavior or conduct with and treatment of individuals are called

    a. DNR.
    b. ethics.
    c. living wills.
    d. heath care proxies.

50. When life-sustaining treatment is withheld or withdrawn (i.e. medication that could prolong the person's life such as a ventilator or feeding tube), this becomes a

    a. legal issue.
    b. donor.
    c. health care proxy.
    d. living will.

51. An oral or written instruction about a person's future medical treatment in case they become unable to speak for themselves is

    a. a non-living donation.
    b. an advance directive.
    c. the Patient Self-Determination Act.
    d. informed consent.

52. The type of advance directive that documents an individual's wishes about medical treatment should they be unable to communicate at the end of life is

    a. living will.
    b. health care proxy.
    c. Five Wishes.
    d. DNR.

53. A document that allows a patient to appoint someone to make decisions about their medical care if they should become incapacitated is a

    a. living will.
    b. health care proxy.
    c. Five Wishes.
    d. DNR.

54. A document that addresses the person's medical, personal, emotional, and spiritual needs and encourages discussing wishes with family and physician is called the

    a. living will.
    b. health care proxy.
    c. Five Wishes.
    d. DNR order.

# CHAPTER 6

# HELPING THE FAMILY MEMBERS COPE

## CHAPTER OBJECTIVE

After completing this chapter, the reader will be able to describe the dimensions of anticipatory mourning; identify reactions of family members after the death of their loved one; learn grief interventions and effective communication techniques for before, during, and after the death; and apply interventions for death notification.

## LEARNING OBJECTIVES

After studying the material in this chapter, the reader will be able to

1. identify the aspects of anticipatory mourning.

2. specify recommendations to help caregivers cope with their emotions before the death of their loved one.

3. indicate interventions that improve death notification communication.

## ANTICIPATORY MOURNING

The term anticipatory grief was first coined by Lindemann in 1944 (Rando, 2000). The term is now called anticipatory mourning. Anticipatory mourning may arise before the actual death in the anticipation of a future loss; it represents a normal form of grief. Anticipatory mourning can occur at any time after a diagnosis is made, and it can occur

in dying patients as well as families. Fulton and Fulton (1971) outlined four aspects of anticipatory mourning for the patient's family.

1. Depression

2. Heightened concern for the terminally ill person

3. Rehearsal of the death

4. Attempts to adjust to the consequences of the death

These four aspects of anticipatory mourning clearly show that after family members learn that a loved one is dying, they are likely to become depressed and worry. They will prepare for the death by reviewing in their minds what they think will happen. They will attempt to imagine what the dying and death experience will be like for their loved one; then they will attempt to adjust to the death by imagining what life will be like after their loved one is dead.

### Six Dimensions

There are six dimensions of anticipatory mourning: perspective, time focus, influencing factors, major sources of adaptational demands, generic operations, and contextual levels (Rando, 2000). The first dimension is the perspective of those involved with the dying. These include the patient, the intimate, the concerned other (which could be a neighbor), and the caregiver. The second dimension, *time focus,* refers to the past, present, and future losses that they may experience. The third dimension, *influencing factors*, relates to the psychological, social, and physiological factors. The fourth dimension is the *major sources of adaptational demands*, which include loss and trauma. The fifth dimension of anticipatory mourning is *generic operations*, which include "grief and mourning, coping, interaction, psychosocial reorganization, planning, balancing conflicting demands, and facilitating an appropriate death" (p. 60). The sixth dimension is *contextual levels*, coping with the dying on an intrapsychic, interpersonal, and systemic level. Rando (2000) notes some of the conflicting demands on the intrapsychic level included the following.

- Holding on to versus letting go of the ill person.

- Planning for life after the death of the loved one versus not wanting to betray the loved one by considering life in his or her absence.

- Experiencing the full intensity of the feelings involved in anticipatory mourning versus trying to avoid becoming overwhelmed.

- Acknowledging the terrible reality and its implications versus trying to maintain some hope.

- Paying sufficient attention to and thinking about what is transpiring and how to cope with it versus wanting to avoid nonproductive ruminating or obsessing.

- Balancing support for the ill person's increased dependency versus supporting the ill person's continued need for autonomy.

- Redistributing family roles and responsibilities versus not wanting to do anything that would call attention to or cause more losses for the ill loved one

(p. 85).

Kalish (1985) notes seven things that can be done to improve the quality of time spent with a dying patient or with a family member who is either experiencing anticipatory mourning or bereavement following a death.

1. Be more conscious of what is going on.

2. Probe your own assumptions and expectations to try to understand how you developed your views.

3. Be honest with yourself about what you are willing to give to the dying or bereaved; otherwise you will find it difficult to be honest with them.

4. Try to understand your own feeling about death and dying. Your own anxieties and denial can limit your competence.

5. Be willing just to be there, without doing anything.

6. Be aware of your energy levels and avoid exhaustion and burnout.

7. Don't try to impose your philosophy of dying or your notion of appropriate grieving on the person you are seeking to help

(p. 268).

# FAMILY TASKS AND REACTIONS

In their study of expectancy and bereavement, Donnelly, Field, and Horowitz (2000-2001) found those with longer terminal illnesses had time to acknowledge and expect death, which lessened the intensity of mourning for their spouse. Martinson (2001) notes, "I thought that if we could get a better understanding of the timing of death, that we as nurses could bring family members in to be with the dying person" (p. 65). She says, "We, as health care professionals, are responsible for creating an environment so the family can function during these valuable hours, day, weeks and, at times, months" (p. 69).

The nurse's primary role is to provide direct nursing care to the terminally ill patient. Bookwala et al. (2001) found that more than 88% of terminally ill individuals in the sample worried they would become dependent and stated that their desire for a dignified death influenced the choices they made concerning their medical treatment. When an individual becomes ill, family members feel stress and that stress comes from the burden of care. Whether it is the isolation they feel or the changes in their roles, they are no longer the same person they were before their loved one became ill. There is also the stress of financial concerns. As the dying patient relies on family members for support, the primary care giver (PCG) has certain perceptions of the situation. Nurses must reevaluate the caregiver and monitor the situation often to intervene and be supportive before a crisis develops (Brinson & Brunk, 2000). Those whose loved ones died because of illness were grateful the suffering was over (Gamino, Hogan, & Sewell, 2002). However, while the patient is alive, the caregiver has the burden of care, and nurses can offer the family a connection to community resources. The resources may support family members who are experiencing anticipatory mourning. Reinhard (2001) notes,

> Nurses need to think of this family as an extension of the person that they are caring for and remember the following principles:

- Nurses need to do some community resource homework to have the telephone numbers of potential supports available.... Families will need ongoing concrete and emotional support. Nurses should expect this need and offer anticipatory guidance.

- Respect all family caregivers. Assume that they are doing the best they can under difficult circumstances. Without their involvement, the client would have fewer options available for ongoing care.

- Give positive reinforcement in all settings. Help identify the strengths that family caregivers have and point them out very concretely. Help them see where they need some assistance—and help them find it.

- Help family caregivers recognize their own needs. Assess family members' needs and capacities

(p. 185).

## Family Grief Interventions Before, During, and After Death

Family treatment begins by understanding what the dying patient, their family members, and health providers want. The Last Acts Task Force on Palliative Care and the Family developed The Five Principles for Better Care at the End of Life (see Figure 6-1). This vision acknowledges the difficulties involved and the hard choices individuals make at the end of life.

Patients who talked about their impending deaths were not more depressed, but the level of relatives' awareness, particularly near the end of their loved one's life, was associated with depression (Hinton, 2003). Nurses help the caregivers cope with their emotions by acknowledging their difficult role. Joan Furman (2001), a nurse, provides ten recommendations to help caregivers cope with their emotions.

1. Build a support system.
2. Allow time for solitude.
3. Keep a sense of humor.
4. Exercise outdoors.
5. Maintain regular interests.
6. Keep a journal.
7. Breathe deeply.
8. Eat well.
9. Find ways to be touched (hugs, massage).
10. Nourish the spirit

(p. 37).

Family caregivers also live with high levels of stress. Furman (2001) points out that nurses can help the family member or caregiver avoid burnout by recommending stress-taming tips:

- Stop negative thoughts about inadequacy as a caregiver by mentally repeating positive thoughts.

- Practice breathing exercises before and after stressful activities by taking 8 or 10

## FIGURE 6-1: A VISION FOR BETTER CARE AT THE END OF LIFE (1 OF 2)

Death and dying are not easy to deal with. Perhaps you or someone you love is facing an illness that cannot be cured. Few of us are really ready for the hard choices that may have to be made at the end of life. It can be hard for everyone involved—the dying person, their family and loved ones, and health care providers, too.

But there are ways to ease pain and make life better for people who are dying and for their loved ones. It is called palliative care. Palliative care means taking care of the whole person—body, mind, spirit—heart and soul. It looks at dying as something natural and personal. The goal of palliative care is that you have the best quality of life you can have during this time.

Some health care providers—doctors, nurses, social workers, pharmacists, clergy, and others - have learned how to five this special kind of care. But all health care providers should know how to give good palliative care or to help find someone who can.

**Five Principles of Palliative Care**

The following Five Principles of Palliative Care describe what care can and should be like for everyone facing the end of life. Some of these ideas may seem simple or just common sense. But all together they give a new and more complete way to look at end-of-life care.

1. *Palliative care represents the goals, like and choices of the dying person. It...*

   Respects your needs and wants as well as those of your family and other loved ones.

   Finds out from you who you want to help plan and give you care.

   Helps you understand your illness and what you can expect in the future.

   Helps you figure out what is important.

   Tries to meet your likes and dislikes: where you get health care, where you want to live, and the kinds of services you want.

   Helps you work together with your health care provider and health plan to solve problems.

2. *Palliative care looks after the medical, emotional, social, and spiritual needs of the dying. It...*

   Knows that dying is an important time for you and your family.

   Offers ways for you to be comfortable and ease pain and other physical discomfort.

   Helps you and your family make needed changes if the illness gets worse.

   Makes sure you are not alone.

   Understands there may be difficulties, fear and painful feelings.

   Gives you the chance to say and do what matters most to you.

   Helps you look back on your life and make peace, even giving you a chance to grow.

3. *Palliative care supports the needs of the family members. It...*

   Understands that families and loved ones need help, too.

   Offers support services to family caregivers, such as time off for rest, and advice and support by telephone.

   Knows that caregiving may put some family members at risk of getting sick themselves. It plans for their special needs.

   Finds ways for family members to cope with the costs of caregiving, like loss of income, and other expenses

   Helps family and loved ones as they grieve.

**FIGURE 6-1: A VISION FOR BETTER CARE AT THE END OF LIFE (2 OF 2)**

4. *Palliative care helps gain access to needed health care providers and appropriate care settings. It...*

Uses many kinds of trained care providers-doctors, nurses, pharmacists, clergy, social workers, and personal care givers.

Makes sure, if necessary, someone is in charge of seeing that your needs are met.

Helps you use hospitals, home care, hospice, and other services, if needed.

Tailors options to the needs of you and your family.

5. *Palliative care builds ways to provide excellent care at the end of life. It...*

Helps care providers learn about the best ways to care for dying people. It gives them the education and support they need.

Works to make sure there are good policies and laws in place.

Seeks funding by private health plans and government agencies.

The Five Principles are a vision for better care at the end of life. They were developed for people who are dying, their families, and their loved ones by the Last Acts task forces on Palliative Care and the Family. Last Acts is a coalition of more than 400 organizations representing health care providers and consumers nationwide.

The organizations involved in last Acts believe that everyone can make a difference in the care given to dying people and their families. We need to work together toward a health care system that offers all Americans, when they are dying:

the services that meet their individual needs

health plans that cover that care

health care providers well trained in palliative care

That would make the Five Principles of Palliative Care a reality.

**What you can do**

You and your family should expect to get good care at the end of life. You can improve the likelihood that you and your family will get the care you want if you:

- Share this document. Discuss the care you want with your family, friends, physicians and other health care professionals, and spiritual advisor. Don't wait until you are seriously ill!

- Learn about your options for care. Make a list of questions to ask your doctor, to find out whether s/he can provide the care you want at the end of life. Visit the Last Acts Web site, www.lastacts.org, for a lit of sample questions.

- Check with your local hospitals, nursing homes, and home health agencies about the special services (palliative care) they offer for dying patients and their families. Examples: Are there physicians, nurses, social workers and spiritual counselors trained in end-of-life care who can talk to you and your family about your concerns? Do you have experts who can manage pain and other physical discomforts? Do they offer bereavement services?

- Find out about local hospice services.

- Think about important decisions now. Prepare a living will and appoint someone to make decisions for you if you are not able (health care proxy).

- Look into community support groups and educational programs for seriously ill patients and their families (often offered by church groups, community centers, libraries and others.

*Source:* Last Acts. *A vision for better care at the end of life.* Available online at http://www.lastacts.org/docs/publicprecepts.pdf

deep breaths while relaxing the body.

- Express feelings by talking, crying, screaming, beating a pillow, or writing.

- Stop setting standards of perfection.

- Resist self-judgment.

- Ask for help.

- Take breaks.

- Write things down to remember them (p. 41).

As the demand for grief-related support has escalated, nurses and health professionals must increase their knowledge of grief and bereavement in order to be effective in providing support to patients and family members. To provide appropriate patient and family care, a fundamental knowledge of the grief process is required. Nurses should be aware of the elements that play a role in the individual's grief. Some of these elements are past grief experiences, personality, social support, type of death, and relationship factors.

## Communication Issues

The role of the family is an important consideration in end-of-life care. Cultural beliefs, customs, and rituals bring comfort to the entire family. Emotional, physical, and spiritual needs of the dying are addressed as clergy and family play a critical role in their care. As the condition of the patient deteriorates, the entire family is affected. Nurses should provide families with options that offer information on various aspects of their loved one's health care. Nurses need to respect the family's beliefs and, in so doing, to be careful not to stereotype the patient in any way. Patients rely on family for guidance and the nurse may have to work with members of the family before any decision is made with respect to terminal care.

The nurse must listen to both the terminally ill patient and the family as they communicate their needs. The nurse must be willing to communicate all options. It is sometimes left to the family to elect cer-

tain procedures for their family member. Therefore, the nurse must remain confident that through this communication, everyone's needs are being met and everyone in the family understands what is being done and not done. The burden of care-giving and financial responsibilities cannot be ignored. All issues must be addressed, as the family's burden creates additional suffering for the terminally ill.

As patients communicate their needs, they take control of their end-of-life care. This begins with devising a plan of action and having an advance directive. The advance directive will enable their wishes to be known when they are no longer capable of communicating those wishes. Communicating one's needs to one's family and health professionals includes discussing issues regarding dying at home or in the hospital, the use of hospice, experiences of anticipatory grief, and the generalized fear of one's own suffering. Complementary therapies and medical pain management can provide the necessary support and comfort to keep patients from turning to suicide.

Effective communication skills begin with knowing what to say as well as knowing what not to say. According to experts examples of what not to say include a variety of standard phrases.

- This must have been God's will.

- At least he/she isn't suffering anymore.

- It was probably for the best.

- I know how you feel.

- You must get a hold of yourself. He/she would want you to.

- At least you have other loved ones.

- It was a good way to go.

- God doesn't give us more than we can bear.

- You'll get over it. Time heals all wounds.

Examples of helpful things to say include more open phrases.

- I'm sorry.

- I'm here if you want to talk.

- How are you doing?

- I don't know what to say.

- I want to help.

- I feel a little bit of your loss.

- I wish I had known him/her better.

- I was sorry to hear about your loss.

- I have great memories of him/her.

- I don't know what to say to be of comfort to you.

- Feel what you feel. (p.97)

> *Personal Insight*
> *What are some phrases you have used that helped a grieving person?*

Communication is much more than talking, it is a learned skill. Communication takes place when information is transferred in a meaningful way. All the topics discussed in this book require some degree of effective communication to succeed. For it to be most effective, the health professional uses simple language, shows concern for any issues raised, pauses, is personal, and allows for ample opportunity to ask questions. To communicate effectively, the nurse must provide an opportunity to discuss choices, share information, offer support, and allow the patient and caregiver to comfortably share their fears. This can be accomplished by using open-ended questions.

- How did you decide that?

- Can you tell me more about how you came to that conclusion?

- Can you explain that to me once again?

- What other alternatives have you thought about?

Reflecting the patient's content and emotion encourages them to share their feelings. As the nurse listens and reflects issues and emotions, the individual will sense that they have been heard. If a patient says, "No one visits me anymore," the nurse can say, "You sound as if you are feeling lonely." If a patient says, "No one is listening to me," the nurse can say, "I really hear you saying that you are frus-

trated." Nurses can reflect a patient's content in a variety of ways.

- I am picking up that you are scared of dying.

- It sounds as if you are most concerned with how your family is coping with your dying.

- I gather that this is hard for you.

- I wonder if you are saying that you want to speak to the clergy.

- If I am hearing you correctly, you do not want to be left alone.

- You sound as if you really do not want any more tests done.

These components of facilitative listening help the patient label his or her emotions. When a patient describes fear of not being given pain medication, the nurse can say, "It sounds as if you are most concerned about being in pain. I will make sure you receive your medication on time." The nurse can find out the most pressing issues for the patient. Verbal messages are just as important as what is not being said. Nurses must be aware of non-verbal messages, such as body language, and take note of posture, eye contact, and facial expressions.

When encouraging conversation, nurses are influenced by their own beliefs and fears regarding their mortality. Nurses who have not experienced the death of a loved one or patient may not be comfortable communicating about death. Nurses may feel extremely uncomfortable speaking with terminally ill patients about the upcoming death. When patients tell their nurse that they just want to die, the nurse may respond by saying, "Oh you really don't mean that." This negates how the patient feels. Nurses who are uneasy may interrupt their patients as they talk about dying and, may attempt to change the subject rather than patiently listening. If nurses are not comfortable sharing emotion, they may also be uncomfortable when tears are shed. Therefore, nurses should explore their own loss issues in order to be better communicators with those who are dying.

If a patient says, "I think that I am going to die soon," or "I just want this over," a nurse can effectively communicate by asking, "What happened today that makes you say this?" Nurses should not attempt to make the patient think about something else. Rather, patients should be encouraged to discuss their own thoughts and feelings. Whether it was something that happened that day or something someone said to them, the matter needs to be addressed and not ignored. Nurses who become comfortable addressing their patient's concerns will provide a great service.

As nurses connect with family members, they can address some of the comments made by insensitive people and the challenge of speaking with insensitive neighbors, friends, and strangers. Furman (2001) notes several such negative statements, "Don't cry. You'll make yourself sick" "See it as a challenge" "Time heals everything" and "She'll be better off dead" (p. 38). Caregivers may also cope with a loved one's terminal illness using humor. They may make light of the situation, and their laughter may help them to cope with the situation. Reasoning and taking one day at a time are other ways caregivers cope with a loved one's illness (Brinson & Brunk, 2000). Nurses should focus on the family and take note of their stress and ability to care for the patient.

Lack of experience with death in the family, sleep deprivation, and physical exhaustion are factors that influence the way a family member will grieve. Family members may feel guilty about not spending enough time with the patient, feel the need to blame someone for their loved one's sickness, feel anger at God for allowing this to happen, or feel fear and worry that the situation will become more than they can bear. Health professionals recognize these feelings are normal and can help the caregiver express such feelings in a healthy way. What is said to the family members will have a direct result on how they cope. Although talking with others helps, it is the nurses and aides who can best describe to the family member any anticipated changes in the foreseeable future. Talking about what will happen will reduce the anxiety when the changes occur.

Placing a terminally ill person in a nursing home is one of the most difficult experiences for the family members. They may rely on the nurse for support, information, and perhaps approval that they are making the right placement decision. If a patient's spouse is considering nursing home placement, a nurse can ask certain questions that may reduce any anxiety.

- "Can you tell me more about how you see your husband's (or wife's) situation?"

- "How did you decide that?"

- "What have you done so far about nursing home placement?"

- "What alternatives have you considered?"

When speaking with family members, the nurse should not use technical language. The family members might not always inform the nurse when they cannot understand what is being said to them. The nurse can ask the family to repeat what they have been told, to confirm what has been discussed. Encourage family members to ask questions. Nonverbal messages communicate to the patient and caregiver that the nurse is interested. These messages include eye contact and facial expression.

McConnell (2001) offers ways nurses can paraphrase and help the person feel as though what they are saying is being understood. "In other words," "You mean," or "Let me see if I understand you" helps the listener feel listened to (p. 74). The nurse should always recognize the role of the caregivers and their valuable contribution to patient care. A nurse can use echoing to facilitate listening. This simple technique opens up discussion. A caregiver may say, "I feel so sad." The nurse can repeat the word in question form, "sad?" The caregiver is encouraged to talk and can then expound on the feelings after the nurse has simply repeated one or a few words from their last sentence.

Effective communication is an essential element in establishing rapport and maintaining any type of interpersonal relationship. Effective communication takes place when understanding has been transmitted from one person to another. Communication can be defined as the ability to understand and be understood. Good communicators appreciate the significance of listening to the whole story and understand the feelings and perceptions of the person sharing the story. In the parable of the horse on the dining room table, the horse in the parable represents death. Neither the host nor the guests make any reference to the horse (see Table 6-2). The host did not want to upset his guests and the guests did not want to upset their host, and so they ate in silence. We cannot ignore death and must learn to acknowledge the horse on our own dining room tables.

The language we use when supporting those who grieve will play a large part in how they cope with their loss. Helping those who grieve is helping them tell their story; in using a narrative, the story of that bond is shared and continued. Hedtke (2002) notes, "I encourage people to speak about their dead partners, to share stories about them, to ask others about what they recalled that they enjoyed about them, and to actively create rituals and celebrations for holidays and anniversaries" (p. 289). Often we are unable to communicate with patients and grieving family members because we have a difficult time communicating about death issues. According to Hogan and Schmidt (2002), "Social support occurs when the bereft believes there is at least one person who will take the time to listen non-judgmentally to them while they openly and honestly express their thoughts and feelings about grief" (p. 619).

The health professional communicates both verbally and nonverbally to establish rapport. Communicating effectively with a person who is dying or one who is grieving is a learned skill. As the patient and nurse communicate, they will explore how hope for a cure becomes hope for other things. Two significant hopes are to complete unfinished business and to be free of pain. Introducing the patient and family to end-of-life care does not mean an end to hope, but it requires the patient to transform that hope.

# DEATH NOTIFICATION

Many professionals encounter difficulties in trying to achieve a positive outcome where providing support to bereaved family members. Rybarik (2000) maintains, "Follow-up phone calls are a challenge for health care providers in several ways: finding time to do the calls, developing the calling in a purposeful manner, and assessing and communicating with patients one cannot see" (p. 224). Professionals can support those who grieve by allowing the individual to view and touch the body, especially if the death came suddenly. Seeing the body helps people accept that their loved one is dead. Touching is an expression of love. After a terminally ill 6-year-old child died, one nurse washed the child and wrapped her in a thick pink blanket. The hospice nurse then tucked in the child's stuffed bunny. She gave the family an opportunity to hold and touch the child. The child's death had a profound effect on the way that nurse practices nursing. The nurse said, "Now I always give family members an opportunity to touch and hold a loved one who died" (Jones, 2001, p. 45). Kavanaugh and Paton (2001) maintain:

> Communication skills are a necessary component of care, but priority is typically not given to learning these skills. In clinical practice, novice clinicians, especially nurses, are often given assignments intended to provide opportunities for increasing technical expertise. Because of this approach, novice nurses often care for infants and parents around the time of a perinatal loss. Yet, as novices, they are typically not prepared to provide time-intensive care of the infant and equally intensive care of the family (p. 376).

A central issue of death notification regarding the health professional's ability to provide support revolves around written communication provided to grieving parents. Reilly-Smorawski, Armstrong, and Catlin (2002) created a contact sheet for bereaved parents to facilitate communication (Table 6-1). This contact sheet offers guidelines for making the initial telephone call after a baby's death. Friedrichs, Daly, and Kavanaugh (2000) noted that after a baby's death, professionals should get the name and sex of the baby, the type of loss, and the date the baby died (p.301). After doing so, the professional is better able to provide phone support to parents after the death of their infant.

Clinicians need to be educated about the behaviors and unique needs of parents after a perinatal loss so their communication becomes a part of caring for the parents (Kavanaugh & Paton, 2001). The primary purpose of communicating with grieving parents is to help them cope during death notification. In understanding the painful experience of losing a child, nurses can provide support by effectively communicating with the parents in a sensitive manner during death notification.

Fauri, Ettner, and Kovacs (2000) noted the following list of recommended specific services that can be used as a guide when hospital staff offer interventions to family survivors.

1. Making immediately available at the time of loss a private, quiet, nicely furnished room as a place for family privacy.

2. Arranging, if desired by the survivor(s), the presence of a chaplain, minister, rabbi, or priest.

3. Arranging for a time and place for a private viewing of the body and for saying goodbye.

4. Providing assistance in obtaining those belongings the deceased brought to the facility.

5. Offering individual, non-directive counseling.

6. Informing survivors of opportunities for participation in support groups.

## TABLE 6-1: GUIDELINES FOR MAKING THE INITIAL TELEPHONE CALL AFTER A BABY'S DEATH

1. Parents should be contacted by their baby's primary nurse 1-3 weeks after the death.

2. The caller should slowly and clearly introduce herself/himself at the outset. The caller must establish that they are speaking with the parent and should mention that they are calling from the hospital.

3. Ask whether this is a good time to talk. (Are there children crying in the background? Are they on their way out?) If this is an inconvenient time, ask when you may call back.

4. Suggested *opening phrases* and *themes* for the discussion:

   A. We generally call families during this difficult time after their child's death to let them know we are thinking of them.

   B. Did you have a memorial service or a ceremony after the baby died?

   C. What was the service like? Did you find it to be a comfort?

   D. Has you partner returned to work?

   E. How much sleep are you getting? Are you troubled by dreams or nightmares?

   F. Are you able to eat?

   G. What have your days been like since the baby's death?

   H. Do you have photographs or a booklet from the time of your baby's death?

      i. Have you been able to look at them?

      ii. Have you been able to share them with others? If so, how have they responded?

   I. What have family/friends done that has been helpful since the baby died?

   J. Who are the support people for you and your partner?

5. If the parents have other children:

   A. How old are your children? How are they reacting to the loss?

   B. May we provide you with information or resources pertinent to sibling grieving?

6. Do you have questions or unresolved issues about the baby's death? Would you like for us to arrange a meeting to discuss these?

*Source:* Reilly-Smorawski, B, Armstrong, A.V. & Catlin, E.A. (2002). Bereavement support for couples following death of a baby: Program development and 14-year exit analysis. *Death Studies, 26*(1), p. 35.

7. Initiating follow-up correspondence with the family concerning hospital records and procedures.

8. Sending flowers or sympathy cards from the institution and its staff to the family at a set period of time after the loss.

9. Placing phone calls to the family as a courtesy and to inquire if further needs or unresolved issues exist.

10. Making referrals to community agencies.

Death notifiers are in a unique position, as what they say and do not say, and what they do and do not do, will have a profound effect of the survivors. The death of a family member is one of life's most difficult moments. Though family reactions will vary from denial to hysteria, the nurse's presence will alleviate many fears. An emergency department nurse explained how she helped the bereaved after a sudden unexpected death.

> Well, I guess I just wait and let the family set the guidelines. You have to judge each family differently. Sometimes your approach works, and sometimes it doesn't... Just kind of say the least amount possible. Just tell them what's happened, and ask if there's anything you can do and so forth. You know, let them either verbalize or not verbalize, and go from there. Some people you have to reassure and talk and talk; and some people, it's best just not to say very much of anything (Iserson, 1999, p. 217).

Informing a survivor that their loved one is dead is not an easy task. Stewart, Lord, and Mercer (2000) note, "Among all respondents, death from a violent interpersonal crime was ranked as placing the most emotional demands on the notifiers when they contacted the survivors" (p. 621). There are several potential barriers to effective death notification. In most cases, the staff in an emergency department does not have a chance to know the family of the deceased. Not knowing the family makes the task of death notification that much more difficult.

## TABLE 6-2: POTENTIAL BARRIERS TO EFFECTIVE EMERGENCY DEPARTMENT NOTIFICATION

- No pre-existing relationship with medical staff.
- Survivor stress: fear, grief, remorse, anxiety, panic.
- Time: staff has limited time, needs to treat other patients/crisis, and may be interrupted to make other decisions.
- Strange environment: Surroundings, noise, smells, lack of privacy.
- Survivor status/behavior: anger, inebriation, disbelief, not available.
- Cultural or language differences.
- Medical staff stress: must deliver bad news, ask for autopsy (or notify about medical examiner requirements), ask for organ/tissue donation, and allow time in the midst of other patients' emergencies.
- Medical staff anger: decedent caused other injuries or deaths.
- Uncertainty: often not clear about the exact cause or manner of death
- Sense of failure: "losing" a patient often pervades discussions

*Source:* Iserson, K.V. (1999). *Grave words: Notifying survivors about sudden, unexpected deaths.* Galen Press, Ltd.: Tucson, AZ.

Those who deliver bad news experience stress along with the survivors. Survivors wait in a strange environment, while the medical staff experiences a sense of failure and stress. These potential barriers are listed in Table 6-2.

When a loved one dies outside the home, family members are notified. It is not recommended that family members be notified by telephone, especially in cases of sudden loss. If at all possible, two qualified personnel in uniform should make notification when going to a survivor's home. After confirming the identity of the family member, the survivor is told that there has been an emergency and that a death has occurred. Parents of murdered children have reported the need to reconstruct the scene. Therefore, when delivering death notification to parents of murdered children, it is important for professionals to provide complete and accurate details of the murder. By providing consistent information, parents will be better equipped to recreate the death scene later on (Dannemiller, 2002).

> Stewart, Lord, and Mercer (2000) point out

> Persons with far less training than mental health professionals in how to respond to acute trauma and loss reactions (e.g., uncontrollable crying) routinely must tell of a death and attempt to help the survivors in their important initial efforts to cope (p. 625).

A likely result of this factor is that the notifiers may not say the right things or provide the necessary support to the survivors, as they do not have the skills to do so effectively. Skills include knowing what to say and how to say it as well as knowing the likely responses of family members. Death notification begins by providing information honestly and clearly. The National Organization of Parents of Murdered Children, Inc. has put together information for doctors and nurses on what is appropriate when informing families or survivors of a loved one's death by violence (see Table 6-3). Professionals benefit from being trained in death notification to help them be compassionate and supportive to the survivors. Stewart et al. (2000) note,

> If notifiers understand how compassion and support can benefit the survivors, they may be less inclined to experience the notification as a guilt-ridden process in which they must "admit defeat" in saving a life (p. 627).

## Four Stages

Iserson (1999) maintains that death notification can be divided into four stages: *Prepare, Inform, Support,* and *Afterwards*. The first stage begins with *Prepare*.

- *Anticipate* the needs of the bereaved by having a room available to speak with them and a room to view the body; know the policies and protocol of your facility before meeting with them.

- *Identify* the person who died, the survivor's name, and the circumstances of death.

- *Notify* the survivor, medical examiner, and patient's physician, and meet them when they arrive.

- *Organize* the groups of survivors; remove them from the corridor into a room; offer drinks, blankets, and tissues; have information regarding any lab tests; and most importantly, organize what you are going to say to the survivors before saying anything.

Iserson identifies *Inform* as the second stage.

- *Introduce* yourself and identify the survivors to make sure you are speaking with the right family.

- *Tell* the survivor what happened — use the decedent's name, use non-technical language, and always use the word "death" or "died." Do not apologize or argue with the survivors; it is okay to show your emotions.

The third stage is *Support*.

- *Reassure* the survivors and assure them that everything was done to save their loved one.

- *Relieve* them, if possible, of any guilt, avoid clichés, and explain some of the common reactions.

- *Assist* them by answering their questions, ask them what they need, help them to make necessary contacts, and provide access to a phone.

- *Answer* questions, even those unasked, by providing written material, including phone numbers and information they may need. Explain how the decedent's clothes and belongs will be returned.

- *Communicate* with clergy if they request it and give them your telephone number so they can communicate with you. If they want to *view* the body, explain any injuries before doing so, and be respectful of their cultural beliefs.

## TABLE 6-3: APPROPRIATE RESPONSE WHEN INFORMING FAMILIES/SURVIVORS OF A LOVED ONE'S DEATH BY VIOLENCE

- Provide a quiet, private area.
- Have a telephone/beverage/restroom, etc. easily accessible.
- If possible, have as many of the family/survivors in the room as possible before informing them of the victim's death.
- Have only one professional speak with the group.
- After introducing yourself, obtain the identity of whom you are addressing to assure the correct family/survivors are in the room.
- Sit with whom you are addressing, do not stand above them.
- Speak face to face with the individual you are addressing, maintaining eye contact.
- Touch the person, such as placing your hand on the person's knee, or holding their hand.
- Speak softly and directly; avoid being "wordy."
- Be up front and timely with what they need to be informed. Family/survivors are understandably impatient in such situations, so lengthy introductions are not appropriate.
- Use the word "dead." It is universally understood. What is suggested is, "I have bad news for you," and then inform them of the victim's death.
- Never use words such as "passed away," "gone to a better place," "with their maker," etc. Such comments are easily misunderstood.
- If the patient is not dead, but death is expected or a possibility, inform the family/survivors the patient is "critical". Inform them of ongoing resuscitation. What is recommended is, "Hope for the best, but be prepared for the worst."
- Be aware of individual and cultural differences regarding the grieving process. Some cultures may respond in a calm manner, while others express anger, disbelief, or respond in a loud, verbal manner.
- Be aware the moment that you are sharing is a moment the family/survivors will never forget. The face and voice of the professional delivering such a message will forever remain in their memory.

- Offer the opportunity to the family/survivors to spend a few moments with the deceased. Prepare them for what they may view, and inform them of why items, such as evidence and medical procedures, may not be removed from the victim's body.
- Provide the opportunity for the family/survivors to contact you if additional information is necessary, or unanswered questions remain. Such a moment is very emotional and confusing, and questions and/or need for additional information may arise during the following days, weeks or months.
- After leaving the family/survivors, return a few moments later to assure all information has been provided, and additional arriving family/survivors have been adequately informed of what has occurred.
- Provide religious/spiritual support, if indicated or requested.
- Explain potential Law Enforcement/Medical Examiner Policies that impact and possibly restrict what will happen to the victim's body.
- Provide assistance regarding funeral arrangements, if requested.
- Do not leave family/survivors alone for extended periods of time. Provide constant visitation from a physician, nurse, social worker, etc., so prompt assistance is available.
- If discussing a patient's status with a family member of friend by telephone, be as honest and clear as possible. Do not provide false optimism. If the patient is dead, and you have documented the identity of the caller, tell the caller the truth.
- If the family/survivors inquire regarding pain and suffering experienced by the victim, make every effort to respond to their questions in a compassionate, honest, thorough, and professional manner. Family/survivors need and want the truth. Therefore, be as straight forward as possible.
- For more information on working with survivors of homicide victims, or to schedule a training session in your area, contact POMC at natlpomc@aol.com or by calling 1.888.818.POMC.

*Source:* The National Organization of Parents Of Murdered Children, Inc. Information for doctors and nurses. Available online at http://www.pomc.com/doctors.cfm

- *Protect* them from the media and be prepared for violent outbursts.

- *Provide* support by arranging for a hotel if they are from out of town.

- *Conclude* by asking if they have any questions, and give them copies of all the papers they signed and the decedent's belongings. Call for someone to take them home if they are alone, and walk them to the exit.

The last stage of Iserson's protocol is *Afterwards*.

- *Debrief* by speaking with staff who participated in the resuscitation, and express your feelings. Tell staff they can release information to callers that the individual has died.

- *Follow-up* the next day with the survivors, ask them if they have any questions, and send a sympathy card.

The way the professional delivers death notification will have a profound effect on the survivor. Throughout the process, bereavement support should be offered. This support can be as simple as placing a warm blanket around the shoulders of a survivor or listening to the bereaved talk about their loss.

Nurses may be called upon to help grieving parents create a memory of their baby. Gensch and Midland (2000) recommend that parents be given the option of holding their baby no matter the gestational age. Other recommendations include taking photos of the infant. After the baby is measured and weighed, the information can be written on a card and placed in a memory box. The baby's I.D band, crib card, sachets of baby powder, and plaster hand or foot prints can be included in the packet that goes home with the grieving parents. The death notifier is in a position to ease the pain of loss by being sensitive to the needs of the bereaved. Ujda and Bendiksen (2000) noted after a perinatal loss, parents found the following particularly unhelpful.

1. Being given a hospital room on the maternity floor where healthy babies could be seen and heard.

2. Lack of communication with the parents during the miscarriage process.

3. Having the supportive person who had accompanied the mother be asked to leave.

4. Being asked to transport the miscarried fetus to the laboratory.

5. Having a dilation and curettage (i.e., a surgical procedure often done with miscarriage) procedure in the emergency room without an anesthetic, without being told what was happening (p. 276).

A nurse may be asked to inform a patient that she is experiencing a miscarriage. The nurse can discuss the procedures being done and the grief the patient may be feeling. To the parents, this is their baby. Though it may be painful for parents to see the fetus, nurses should ask them if they want to see it. Ujda and Bendiksen (2000) maintain,

Besides choosing their words carefully and with sensitivity, health care providers can contribute to their parent's feelings of being well cared for if they:

- simply say how sorry they are;

- avoid minimizing even the earliest loss, treating baby or fetus with respect;

- avoid using the word *common* to describe the parents' loss experience;

- offer all parents with perinatal loss written information about their loss and about the availability of bereavement resources and counseling; and

- learn to assess the patient's coping resources and recognize symptoms such as prior depression and lack of social support that signal the possibility of chronic grief development (p. 280).

Once death notification is made, the grieving individual begins the process of coping with their loss.

> *Personal Insight*
> *If you had to deliver bad news, what did you say? How did the person respond to what you were saying? How did their response make you feel?*

# SUMMARY

This chapter examined some of the major issues facing the family of the dying patient. By explaining the concept of anticipatory mourning, the four aspects of anticipatory mourning for the patient's family—depression, heightened concern for the terminally ill person, rehearsal of the death, and attempts to adjust to the consequences of the death—were reviewed. Six dimensions of anticipatory mourning were highlighted; perspective, time focus, influencing factors, major sources of adaptational demands, generic operations, and contextual levels.

Within this chapter, family tasks and reactions and the nurse's primary role as providing direct nursing care to the terminally ill patient were explored. Family treatment interventions before, during, and after death were highlighted. The Five Principles for Better Care at the End of Life were explored. In this chapter, ten recommendations were offered to help caregivers cope with their emotions, and ways nurses can help the caregiver avoid burnout by recommending stress-taming tips were noted. The health professional's providing written communication to grieving parents and the need for clinicians to be educated about the behaviors and unique needs of parents after a perinatal loss were examined. A list of recommended specific services that can be used as a guide when hospital staff offer interventions to family survivors was included.

This chapter included a list of things that can be done to improve the quality of time spent with a dying patient or a family member who is experiencing anticipatory grief or bereavement. Near the end of this chapter, the importance of effective communication was stressed. Nurses are influenced by their beliefs and fears regarding their own mortality, so we discussed ways nurses can become comfortable addressing their patient's concerns about death, dying, and bereavement.

The chapter ended with the unique position of the death notifier, one who informs survivors that their loved one is dead. The four stages of death notification and the protocol for sudden-death notification were examined. Ways the death notifier can ease the pain of loss by being sensitive to the needs of the bereaved were discussed.

# RESOURCES

## Helping the Family Member Cope on the Internet

Alzheimer's Disease and Related Disorders
    Association
    www.alz.org

Genetic Alliance (formerly The Alliance of
    Genetic Support Groups)
    www.geneticalliance.org

Hospice Foundation of America
    www.hospicefoundation.org

National Self-Help Clearinghouse
    www.selfhelpweb.org

# EXAM QUESTIONS

## CHAPTER 6
### Questions 55-65

55. The process of mourning that may arise before the actual death is best characterized as

    a. family tasks.
    b. complicated.
    c. anticipatory.
    d. palliative.

56. The first dimension of anticipatory mourning involves the

    a. patient, the intimate, and the concerned other.
    b. past, present, and future losses.
    c. psychological, social, and physiological factors.
    d. major sources of adaptational demands.

57. The fourth dimension of anticipatory mourning involves

    a. patient, the intimate, and the concerned other.
    b. past, present, and future losses.
    c. psychological, social, and physiological factors.
    d. major sources of adaptational demands.

58. A recommendation to help caregivers cope with their emotions is to

    a. mentally repeat the negative thoughts.
    b. attempt standards of perfection.
    c. ignore regular interests.
    d. find ways to be touched.

59. After a baby's death, the baby's primary nurse should make the initial telephone call to the parents

    a. 1-3 weeks later.
    b. 3-6 weeks later.
    c. 3 months later.
    d. 6 months later.

60. One guideline for nurses making the initial telephone call after a baby's death is

    a. not to ask if parents have questions or unresolved issues.
    b. to slowly and clearly introduce yourself at the outset.
    c. inform the parents that no meetings will be arranged.
    d. speak with anyone who answers.

61. An opening phrase used when following the guidelines for callers making the initial telephone call after a baby's death is

    a. "we generally call families during this difficult time to let them know how difficult it is for us to make this call."
    b. "we do not feel the need to discuss the memorial service or a ceremony after your baby died."
    c. "we know you must not be sleeping and having nightmares."
    d. "do you have photographs or a booklet from the time of your baby's death?"

62. After a baby's death, professionals should

    a. get the name and sex of the baby.

    b. attempt to make the parents move on with their life.

    c. not allow the parents to hold and touch the child.

    c. discard any belongings of the infant.

63. According to Iserson, the four stages of death notification are

    a. prepare, inform, assist, protect.

    b. prepare, anticipate, debrief, follow-up.

    c. prepare, inform, support, afterwards.

    d. prepare, protect, provide, conclude.

64. To prepare for death notification, the notifier should

    a. reassure the survivors.

    b. anticipate the needs of the bereaved.

    c. follow-up the next day.

    d. answer questions, even those unasked.

65. According to Iserson, during the *Inform* stage, a death notifier should

    a. communicate with clergy if they request it.

    b. protect them from the media and be prepared for violent outbursts.

    c. use the decedent's name and use non-technical language.

    d. arrange for a hotel if they are from out of town.

# CHAPTER 7

# LIFE SPAN ISSUES

## CHAPTER OBJECTIVE

After completing this chapter, the reader will be able to describe life span issues facing grieving children, adolescents, adults, and the elderly.

## LEARNING OBJECTIVES

After studying the material in this chapter, the reader will be able to

1. specify children's and adolescent's understanding of death.

2. recognize how interventions with bereaved children and adolescents lead to coping with loss.

3. identify the most common and difficult adjustments for grieving older adults

4. recognize responses found in grieving adults.

## CHILDREN AND ADOLESCENTS

### Encounters with Death and Bereavement

Loss is experienced through an entire life span, beginning in childhood. Whether the loss is a person, place, or object, it is meaningful to the individual. For children, the meaning of their losses will change as they age, and they will continue to rework the pain. In helping children and adolescents develop a healthy orientation toward death, adults in their life model certain behaviors. Adults should be honest with children and adolescents about death and not attempt to conceal their emotions. During this difficult time, adults and children can come together and share their fears.

Yang and Chen (2002) found that some children reported feeling anxious about the great deal of pain their loved one might feel as they approach imminent death. Some children report being afraid the dead will come back as ghosts. The authors found that most children's fear of death is related to their fear of being permanently separated from their loved one. The children reported feeling anxiety because of this separation and being unable to finish what they wanted to do after their loved one died. Adults can alleviate fears by discussing pain management. Adults can also explain what happens to the body as one dies and talk about beliefs about afterlife. They can talk about the transition, what happens to the body once a person dies, and fears, including fears of ghosts.

Though it is common for children between the ages of 3 and 5 to think of a person who has died as a ghost, it is also possible for older children to believe their loved one will be coming back as a ghost. This may reflect cultural beliefs. Fear of separation can be addressed by helping the child continue the bond with their loved one. Though the person is dead, a child can form a spiritual bond with them. Silverman, Nickman, and Worden (1995)

115

found five categories that reflect a child's efforts to maintain a connection to the deceased parent.

1. Making an effort to locate the deceased (ie. heaven).

2. Actually experiencing the deceased in some way.

3. Reaching out to initiate a connection (ie. visiting cemetery).

4. Remembering.

5. Keeping something that belonged to the deceased (p. 137).

Children and adolescents experience a variety of losses. These may include losing a pet, divorcing parents, moving to a new school, missing a friend who moved away, and mourning a grandparent's death. Each of these losses will add to the child's understanding of death, dying, and bereavement. Sometimes the child may appear unaffected, as he or she might not understand the permanence of death or its meaning. However, as the child ages, the permanence of the death becomes more evident.

## Children's Understanding of Death

Though infants and toddlers may perceive that adults are sad or distraught, children this young have no real understanding of the meaning of death. The perceptions of children between the ages of 2 and 4 are modeled after their parent's behavior. Children understand the concept of death by the age of 3; to them death is a separation and not a permanent situation. Between the ages of 3 and 5, children focus on their own needs first. They want to know who will take care of them. If a child's mother was killed in a car accident, one of the child's first questions might be, "Who is going to make me peanut butter sandwiches?" Though denial is likely, they may believe that their loved one is going to come back to life. When explaining death to a child in this age group, it is best to explain the death in physical terms (ie. the heart stops beating). The child may even wonder what the deceased is doing. Death is confusing, and the child may be scared. If the child appears cranky,

adults may see the child's feelings acted out through play. Though children between the ages of 3 and 5 are fascinated with dead things (such as dead insects or dead animals on the side of the road), they may act as if their loved one did not die. Before the age of 5, children do not see death as irreversible. In their minds, the dead person continues to exist.

Between the ages of 5 and 9, children understand that when a person dies, they cannot come back to life, that death happens to everyone, and that when you die your body stops working. By this age, children begin to understand the finality of death. The five most frequently examined aspects of children's understanding of death are non-functionality, irreversibility, universality, causality, and personal mortality, with most children understanding all of the components by about 10 years of age (Speece & Brent, 1984).

1. Non-functionality refers to the understanding that all life-sustaining functions cease with death.

2. Irreversibility refers to the understanding that death is final and, once dead, a person cannot become alive again.

3. Universality refers to understanding that death is inevitable to living things and that all living things die.

4. Causality refers to understanding what causes death.

5. Personal mortality is related to universality but reflective of the deeper understanding not only that all living things die, but that "I will die"
(p. 65).

---

***Personal Insight***
*What are your earliest memories of death? Was it a friend, pet, or family member who died? What did people say to you after the death?*

---

Children age 5 to 9 give death a personality. The term "boogieman" is a common euphemism for death in this age group. As children in this age group ask questions about death, adults should be open and honest as they attempt to answer the often-difficult questions. Children fluctuate from showing no emotion and playing as usual to showing a great deal of emotion as they seek answers. If a family member died at home, it is not uncommon for children in this age group to not want to go into the room where their loved one died. Children may feel sad, anxious, or withdrawn and may experience nightmares as they attempt to understand death.

Children over the age of 9 generally understand the concept of death, as shown in the following example.

**Example**

John worked as an LPN in an urban hospital and was caring for a 42-year-old female with heart disease. The patient's 10-year-old daughter, Fran, visited often. John overheard Fran's aunt tell the child that her mother would be fine, even though the patient was actively dying. A few days prior, John had been in the patient's room when Fran attempted to discuss her mother's dying with a family friend who was visiting. Fran had been told not to talk about her mother's sickness in front of the patient because that would make her mother very sick. Fran had recently had a cold and asked if her mom was sick because she had caught her cold. The friend told her that it was not her fault and that her mom was suffering from a heart condition. Later the friend and the patient's husband were discussing funeral arrangements and choice of caskets. Fran asked if she should draw a picture of herself and her mother to put into the casket. The friend rejected the suggestion. However, Fran's father told her that he thought her mom would appreciate the drawing. The family friend then asked John if he thought it was a good idea for Fran to

put a picture in the patient's casket. John told him that it is important to involve children in funeral planning. He recommended asking Fran to draw a picture or place a photograph in the casket. Fran's mom had been buying Fran's hair ornaments for years, so Fran's dad thought placing a few of Fran's hair ribbons in his wife's hand would be special. John told him that putting these special small objects into the casket would help to involve Fran and make her feel important. The nurse also told the father that he had overheard a family friend tell Fran that she should not talk about her mother's illness in front of her mother. The nurse recommended that Fran be given permission to talk about her mother's terminal illness with her mom, explaining the importance of listening to Fran and being honest with her about her mother's condition.

Though children understand the finality of death, it is still difficult to discuss. They may act out and find it difficult to concentrate or sleep. They may feel lonely and abandoned or act as if the death never happened. Children in this age group may believe that they caused their special person to die. Adults must continually reinforce that the death was not caused by something the child did or did not do. The child may experience nightmares and behave aggressively as he or she copes with the pain of loss.

Lisa Murphy, a staff nurse at Blessing Hospital in Illinois, was caring for a female in her thirties who was dying of cancer. The nurse attempted to explain to the patient's 9-year-old son that his mother was dying. The nurse knelt down to his eye level and softly said, "This is what dying is, Jay. Your mommy is dying. She doesn't want to, but she can't help it and she can't stop it....Your mommy can't talk with you now, but she can hear you...She can't reach out and hug you, but she can feel you touch her." The nurse put the child on the bed next to his mother and held his hand. He cried and asked, "Mommy are you sleeping?... Mommy, Mommy don't leave me. I promise I'll be a good boy. I promise I'll do better in school." His mother could not respond and before jumping off the bed and running out of the room into his father's arms, he said, "Mommy, I love you." (Murphy, 2001, p. 62)

The nurse understood the child's concept of death and how difficult it was for him to understand at his young age. The nurse used the word "dying" and assured him that his mother did not want to leave him. She also spoke to him at his eye level and reassured him that even though his mother could not speak, she could hear what he needed to tell her. Before running out of the room, his last words to his mother were, "Mommy I love you." Because of what the nurse said, this child would always know that his mother heard him.

The advice and information provided by nurses and health care professionals can help the entire family cope with a loss. Grieving adults may ask the nurse whether or not a child should be allowed to go to the funeral home. This answer is simple...as long as the child is prepared and wants to go. Preparing a child begins by explaining that after someone dies, the body is taken to a place called a funeral home and that the body will stay there until the burial. Everything that the child will see at the funeral home should be explained. This includes the casket, the color of the clothes the deceased will be wearing, the flowers, and the mourners present. If the adult has been to the funeral home before, they can explain the color of the rug as well as the paintings on the wall. This familiarizes the child with what he or she will see and comforts them in a stressful situation.

After preparing the child for what he or she will see at the funeral home, ask if they want to go. No matter what the age of the child, they should be allowed to make their own choices as to whether or not they want to attend the funeral. As adults provide

information, children will be better able to make the decision about whether or not they want to attend.

> **Personal Insight**
> *How old were you when you first attended a funeral? What was the experience like for you?*

## Identifying and Assessing the Bereaved Child

After the death of a loved one, the bereaved child will move in and out of grief. Each child is an individual and will react to the loss differently. As we identify grieving children and assess their needs, we must look at how the significant adult in their life is coping with the loss. If a parent is unable to cope with the loss and is experiencing anxiety, they may have difficulty talking with the child. By addressing the anxiety a parent feels, the child's anxiety can be lessened.

Common emotional grief reactions in children include being numb, sad, withdrawn, angry, self-blaming, helpless, and silly. Mental reactions include impaired concentration, preoccupation, nightmares, and sleep disturbances. Some of the physical reactions are changes in appetite, stomachaches, bladder and/or bowel changes, rashes, headaches, and breathing disturbances. Behavioral reactions include clinging, hoarding toys, and being defiant, as well as self-destructive behaviors. Aggressive behavior might mask depression. Children's depression is often not what we expect to see. We may assume that the grieving child would be sad and sit in a chair, not eat or be able to sleep. Though this happens, grieving children who are depressed can be aggressive, hyperactive, and inattentive. A bereaved child may experience a spiritual reaction where they feel judged by God, disconnected, lost, and empty. They may also feel the presence of the one who died.

Several factors may complicate identifying and assessing the bereaved child. These factors include the type of death, the child's characteristics, social support, and multiple losses (Williams, Hackworth, & Cradock, 2002). If the death was sudden or stigmatized, as in the case of suicide, the child may not feel comfortable talking about the loss. If the child is shy and does not have friends to talk to, this may complicate the grief process. Factors that may complicate grief include multiple losses, death of both parents, and deaths of other significant people in their life.

## Interventions with Bereaved Children

Just thinking about talking to children about death can make health professionals nervous. While offering prompt and accurate information to bereaved children, nurses should speak with them in age-appropriate words and tell them what happened. Consider, for example, a female patient who died at the hospital. Immediately after her death, her 7-year-old daughter was told by the father that her mother was at rest. The child walked over to her mother's nurse and asked if her mother was sleeping. The nurse told her that after a person sleeps, they feel rested, but that when a person dies, the body does not work anymore. The nurse explained that some people say "at rest" or "at peace" when they really mean "dead." The nurse offered emotional support, reassuring her that her mother was not resting and that she would not wake up. The nurse also spoke with the child's father and focused on the child's needs, reviewing what happens to the body when a person dies. He could then model the dialogue and share the same information with his daughter if she should ask him the same question.

Bereaved children grieve in a family context. As families attempt to cope with the loss, children may become depressed and frightened. They may ask the same questions repeatedly. Health professionals may advise adults to answer the child honestly as the child attempts to make sense of the loss. The questions help them understand what happened. Adults should continue to encourage children to ask questions. One helpful intervention with bereaved

children is to hold and rock them. Encourage the child to maintain an attachment to the deceased.

Nurses can help children share stories and experiences. In such sharing, children attempt to understand that their loved one is dead. Nurses can help grieving adults talk to their child about their feelings and recommend rituals they can do together. Through these rituals of remembrance, the child can more easily incorporate the loss. Fox (1988) described children's tasks in coping with loss and grief. Corr modified these tasks (1995) noting that they are:

a) to understand and begin to make sense out of what has happened;

b) to identify, validate, and express in constructive ways their strong reactions to the loss;

c) to commemorate the life that was lived; and

d) to learn to go on with living and loving (p. 14).

Linking objects are items that once belonged to the deceased that the child now owns. In taking ownership of a linking object, the significance of the item becomes very important. Rubel (1999c) points out some questions and ideas that adults can explore with the child regarding linking objects.

- Do I have something that belonged to my special person? If so, describe it.

- If I could have one item that belonged to my special person, what would it be?

- Draw a picture of something that belonged to my special person.

- Why does the object have special meaning?

- Am I doing anything with my special person's object?

- How does the object make me feel connected to my special person?

- How would I feel if the object was lost? (p. 15).

As a child learns to go on living and loving the person who died, it is up to the adults to help them do so. Nurses can advise the adults in the child's life to offer the child something that belonged to their special person.

## Adolescents' Understanding of Death

Though individuals between the ages of 10 and 21 have been referred to as adolescent, this text shall refer to adolescence as the period from 14 to 19 years of age. Early adolescence (roughly ages 10 to 14) is a monumental time in the life of a child. They are worrying about their appearance, experiencing hormonal changes, and asserting their independence. During this time, most adolescents experience the onset of puberty. Friends become very important, and they want to identify as closely as possible with their friends. Their siblings are also significant; losing a sibling during this time can shatter their world.

> Chris was an early adolescent (age 13) when her brother died in a freakish motorboat accident. When asked how she responded in the first few weeks following his death, Chris recalled, "I felt like my life was just shattered. It was like this big jolt in my life, and I felt really little compared to the whole world. I had this feeling I was so empty inside. I hurt so bad, going numb was the only way to deal with it" (Balk & Corr, 1996, p. 9).

Middle adolescent (roughly age 15 to 16) boys and girls will change their appearance frequently, become more sociable, and spend less time with family and more time with friends. Late adolescence (roughly ages 17 to 19) brings the teenager into relationships that may become sexual in nature with a boyfriend or girlfriend. Whether early, middle, or late adolescence, young people will rely on relationships to help them cope with issues related to loss.

Noppe and Noppe (1996) point out that adolescents in particular may be vulnerable to conflicting tensions that distinguish their interpretations of death from those of adults. The authors noted that grieving adolescents often took unnecessary risks with their body. Rationality and romanticism, social life and

death, and breaking of the bonds were conflicting tensions also noted. Some adolescents are away at college or making career choices. This is the point where individuals achieve separation from their parents or caregivers. However, it can also be the point where they take unnecessary risks and may not seek out the support of peers or adults in their life.

Lohan and Murphy (2000-2001) studied parents' perceptions of their adolescent child's grief response after their other child, who was also an adolescent or young adult, was suddenly and violently killed. Lohan and Murphy found parents reported shared categories of concerns for their surviving children. Shared themes were:

a) affective responses,

b) struggling to make meaning,

c) existential concerns,

d) interpersonal/social concerns,

e) avoiding and pushing the death away, and

f) the void left behind,

g) filling the shoes,

h) work, school, and sleep problems,

i) physical symptoms,

j) cognitive and communication changes,

k) family relationship and spirituality issues,

l) pregnancy (in a daughter), and

m) positive steps.

Some of the affective responses reported were "sadness," "easily upset," "holding his feelings in," and "anxiety." Some of the struggling to make meaning themes included "hard to go on," "anticipating the future," and "wondering what would have been." Existential concerns reported were "will not live past 30—he just knows it" and "less social without his brother." Examples of the avoidance theme were "not accepting it," "won't talk about it," and "gets upset when sister is discussed." The void left behind concerns included "lost his best friend," "feeling he left her," and "missing at wedding." Examples of filling the shoes were "wear brother's clothes" and "pained by comparisons with sister." A family issue reported was "hard to see parents in pain." Spiritual issues reported were "avoids religion" and "using an Ouija board." An example of a positive step was "accepting" (Lohan & Murphy, 2000-2001).

## Interventions with Bereaved Adolescents

As a nurse, you may be called upon to help a bereaved adolescent. When a child or adolescent experiences the death of a special person, tell them what happened in age-appropriate words. Offer reassurance that their feelings are normal. Inform them about where the body of their loved one has been taken. Adults should not assume adolescents know about funeral homes or customs surrounding death. Advise the adults in the child's life to review the customs and traditions of their faith and culture and involve them in the planning of the funeral and services. Adolescents should be encouraged to talk about their loss.

As nurses provide support, adolescents will share their story, focus on the reality of the death, and start to work out what it means to them. Professionals assisting grieving adolescents must look at their needs within the context of their family system and how others in the family are coping with the loss. Professionals use the following suggestions for assisting adolescents who are coping with death and bereavement.

- Use the words death, suicide, murdered, etc., to let them know they can use these words.
- Identify the person who died and the nature of the relationship.
- Review hospital records.
- Ask where they were when the person died.
- Ask them what happened and the timeliness of the death.
- Identify the most significant problems.

- Identify linking objects that belonged to the deceased that the adolescent may now own.
- Look at pictures of the deceased.
- Review obituaries and/or newspaper articles about the death.
- Explore whether or not they need to hide their feelings.
- Identify previous losses and how they grieved in the past.
- Show concern.
- Draw a family genogram and discuss the relationship of each person included.
- Use guided imagery.
- Review death certificates.
- If possible, visit the grave site together and/or the place of the death.
- Encourage them to ask questions.

Encourage them to let others know what they need, especially if their feelings are ambivalent, guilty, or hostile.

In cases where feelings of ambivalence, guilt, or hostility are expressed in conjunction with feelings of sadness and loss, it might be helpful to coach an adolescent in the expression of these feelings and in the expression of words that were never said or questions that were never asked. These questions and feeling can be shared with other family members as well as directly with the deceased. This can be facilitated by asking the adolescent to write a letter to the deceased person and to express in it whatever 'unfinished' things are still distressing him or her. Rituals such as sending the letter, reading the letter at the grave site, talking to the deceased in an empty chair, or visiting the grave site can be used as a means to express remaining thoughts and feelings (Valentine, 1997, p. 326).

Death impacts an adolescent's school performance and self-esteem (Fleming & Balmer, 1996). Though adolescents can maintain their grades after the death of a significant person, parents and professionals need to be aware of the adolescent's grief as he or she attempts to maintain their grades. Their peers may not know how to respond to them, and adults may assume they are not grieving. Adolescents were attached to their loved one and are attempting to cope with the loss. However, at a time when they need the support of peers and family, they avoid communicating that need. Tyson-Rawson (1997) notes, "Support from family and peers that communicates validation of a bereaved adolescent's experiences and self is a critical element in the resolution of bereavement and the recreation of an effective internal working model of attachments" (p. 165).

The child's or adolescent's self-concept changes after the death of a special person. The way they viewed themselves prior to the loss is not the same way they look at themselves after the loss. Their self-confidence might be lowered as well as their self-esteem. Though friends are very significant and can be supportive in their own way, adults, through their honest and open communication and sharing, are most effective in providing support to adolescents. The child will then decide how much information to share with his friends. When helping bereaved adolescents, adults should remember to provide information honestly and talk with them about what they are feeling. The grieving adolescent may feel shock or guilt and even have thoughts of suicide. They will need to talk about the death and their feelings associated with that loss.

As adults share their own pain of loss, adolescents will find it easier to share their grief. As health professionals reach out to grieving adolescents, they will establish a relationship with them. Adolescents can be resilient as they cope with loss. The adults in their life can provide a good support system through hospices, schools, and faith communities, which

can provide bereavement assistance. Adolescents should be allowed to be with the dying person, attend the funeral, and partake in family rituals. If the death was sudden, and the child did not have the opportunity to say goodbye, as in the case of Alex, a character in *But I Didn't Say Goodbye*, there are still healing rituals in which they can partake (see Figure 7-1).

When helping bereaved children or adolescents, nurses may feel at a loss for words. If this should happen, you can use the following opening sentences as a guide to providing support.

- Tell me about your special person.

- Where were you when your special person died?

- What happened when you heard your special person was dead?

- Is there anything you would have like to have told your special person?

- What do you think happens after death?

# ADULTS

## Adults View Their Childhood Bereavement Experiences

Dickinson, Leming, and Mermann (1994) conducted a study of 440 students enrolled in a death and dying class to determine what they recall about their first childhood death experience. According to Dickinson, a child's death experiences may turn out to be lasting memories for the adult. Most of the students were female and approximately 23 years old. The average age at their first death experience was 7.95. He found that the death of relatives, mostly grandparents, and pets, specifically dogs and cats, were most frequently reported. The participants in the study reported feeling relief, confusion, fear, happiness, anger, sadness, guilt, emptiness, and shock after a death. Crying was the most reported response. In the case of a sudden loss, disbelief was the most reported response. The explanation of

## FIGURE 7-1: BUT I DIDN'T SAY GOODBYE

"My mom said that we were grieving, but we were grieving together. Even though my dad died, we were still a family. And as a family we went to my dad's funeral. I had never been to a funeral before and had no idea what to expect. I think kids should decide if they want to go or not, but need to know from adults what they're like. My dad's body was buried at the funeral. It took place at a cemetery. After the funeral, our family went back to my house. One of the things we did as a family was light a candle and say a prayer. It's important to only light candles when adults are with you. My sister and I would light our own candle after our mom lit hers. My mom then recited a poem. We did this a lot right after Dad died. Now we do it once a year on the anniversary of his death. My mom calls it "our ritual."

I remember one thing I did after my dad died was make a memory book of him. I put photographs of him in it. I also drew many pictures. One of the pictures I drew was of what I thought my dad's death looked like in the basement. I drew him holding a gun to his head. The gun was so big. It was bigger than his body. I also drew tears in his eyes. I showed the picture to my mom and we talked about what she saw after he died.

One of the things I did a few weeks after my dad died was make a collage. I cut things from magazines my dad liked and glued them to a large sheet of paper. I also wrote a story about him. I drew a picture of a time machine too. I imagined a time when my dad was alive. I even drew a picture of my family's wishing well and wrote down all my wishes. It was a neat picture. Mom and my sister also wrote down their wishes.

At first, I wished that I didn't have to go to the support group. But, looking back at it now, I am glad my mom told me to go. It really helped me understand what I was feeling. The kids in the group were nice. I liked drawing with them and talking to them. It made me realize that I wasn't the only one who had a special person die. Some of the kids brought in things that belonged to their special person. I remember one girl wore the necklace of her mom, who died.

I still wear my dad's T-shirt and baseball cap. It feels good having stuff that belonged to my dad. I still have the note I wrote after he died. I let my grandma read the note and we talked about it. She told me stories about when he was a boy and brought me a photo album filled with pictures of him as a kid. It was so cool to see my dad and uncle Sammy as boys.

Grandma told me that I looked just like my dad in one of the pictures. That's the one that I took out of the album and kept on my table in my room. My room has changed since my dad died, five years ago. But, his picture is still on my table. Whatever death is, my dad would never be completely gone. My dad's dead, but he is still a big part of my life and always will be.

I was only ten when he died and really into baseball back then. It was hard not having him take me to the games, but the coach was a big help. I remember the coach took me to a practice a few days after the funeral. I thought everyone would be really weird. But no one on the team mentioned anything about it except for a few of my friends, who said they were sorry my dad died. I really missed my dad at the games. Every time I won a trophy I wished he was there. I think he somehow knows I won the trophy and is proud of me.

I just started taking karate. Is there something you're doing now that your special person would be proud of? Write about it! Think about things you did together. Share your memories and ask your questions. Even now, years after the death, I still ask questions, different ones, all the times. Sometimes I can't figure out the answers. Maybe you're thinking of the same questions or have different ones of your own. I found some answers in books that I have read written for kids who have lost a special person. In the beginning, it was hard to concentrate on anything. As time passed, it was easier to read and learn about what I was feeling. Some of the books had pages in them where I drew and wrote how I felt. I still have the workbooks and sometimes I look back on my pictures and notes. I think that my family, some of my friends, the support group I attended, prayer, and the stuff I read really helped me cope with my dad's death."

*Source:* Rubel, B. (1999c). *But I Didn't Say Goodbye: For Parents and Professionals Helping Child Suicide Survivors.* Kendall Park, NJ: Griefwork Center, Inc. p. 35-37.

death most often reported was that the deceased went to heaven. Many respondents reported traumatic experiences, which included being forced to kiss a deceased relative, watching a pet cat die, and having to wash a dead sister's body before the funeral director came to take the body. A commonly mentioned recollection of funerals was that the deceased looked asleep.

> *Personal Insight*
> *Was death talked about in your family when you were a child? Which member of your family talked with you about death?*

## Encounters with Death and Bereavement

There comes a time in most lives when people think of their own mortality. At this point, the individual reflects on the number of years left to live rather than the time spent. During adulthood, the person grows older and the body physically deteriorates. Each year the person can see himself or herself getting closer to their death.

As individuals age, they reflect on their own lives and the lives of those who were a part of their lives. Adults, at a certain point, know someone who died. Whenever that occurs, the loss affects them in some way or another. The death of a loved one or significant other is an event that customarily initiates the grief process, a multitude of complex responses that follow separation and loss. Grief will be more intense for those bereaved after a traumatic death, especially if the deceased was young and the death seemed preventable (Gamino, Sewell, & Easterling, 2000).

> Give sorrow words. The grief that does not speak whispers the o'erfraught heart and bids it break.  — Shakespeare, *Macbeth*, IV.iii.

The grieving adult's story is shaped by the relationship they shared with the person who died. Gilbert (2002) notes, "Our stories inform our lives and our lives, in turn, are shaped by our stories" (p. 236). As the bereaved share their story and their

pain, their lives are forever changed. When the death is expected, the bereaved experiences anticipatory grief, where he or she completes unfinished business, prepares for the loss, and gradually grasps the certainty that their loved one will die (Straub & Roberts, 2001). In bereavement situations where there is no warning, as in the aftermath of the September 2001 terror attacks, the world of the bereaved is shattered. No matter what the type of loss, those left behind feel the absence. Gamino et al. (2002) note that loved ones experience a "lack of everyday companionship; removal of role interdependence; loss of an anticipated future; an inner void that included even a loss of part of self; and an awful sense of finality and permanence" (p. 809).

When a friend or family member leaves for work, one does not expect that they will not return. Some 5,430 Americans died from injuries suffered while at work. Loss is more difficult to accept when it is sudden. Deaths due to suicides or homicides, multiples deaths, shocking or grotesque deaths, and children's deaths especially shatter the lives of the survivors (Sanders, 2001). Nurses play an important part in the life of the survivors, from attempting to save their loved one's lives to delivering bad news.

> *Personal Insight*
> *Describe a time when you experienced a death of a significant person in your life. What reactions did you have to the death?*

### Death of a Parent

A daughter said,

Sometimes when I'm in the kitchen, I'll say, "Mom, you're right, it's cold in this kitchen." She used to say this is the coldest kitchen. So, I have a tendency to talk to her like that. I don't expect an answer or anything. I just talk to her (Smith, 2002, p. 321).

In speaking with her mother, the bond they shared and their relationship continue after death. There is symbolic meaning in the death of a parent, that does not end in death. It is normal for children to continue speaking with their deceased parent, even when they are no longer physically there.

## Death of a Spouse

In studying the death of a spouse, thanatologists attempt to understand ways that widows remain emotionally and spiritually attached to the deceased. Silverman (2001) suggested the most common ways are through

a) remembering the deceased,

b) talking about the deceased,

c) dreaming about the deceased, and

d) participating in religious and other rituals that honor the dead.

Though remembering, talking, dreaming, and participating in rituals may maintain the bond with the deceased, there are practical matters that grieving individuals must address. Benight, Flores, and Tashiro (2001) note:

> Another client may feel totally incapable of managing the household finances since her husband's death. This client would benefit from consultation with a financial planner, or if the problem is within the expertise of the therapist, the therapist can begin specific skill-building work both with and outside of the therapeutic hour (p.117).

While providing emotional support, a nurse may also address practical matters and offer advice and referrals. As widows develop new roles, they remember and feel connected to the person who died. Nurses can remind those spouses that even though their loved one is dead, their relationship is forever, as cited in the following example.

## Example

Ellen has been working in a short-stay surgical ward for 2 years as a nurse. One morning a patient died suddenly; though Ellen had never experienced a patient's dying before, she was effective in providing emotional support to the patient's spouse. Ellen held her hand and discussed the complications after the routine surgery. She gave the patient's wife permission to talk about him and how he will always be a part of her. Ellen also asked her about her religion and rituals that would honor him, which also provided comfort.

As the bereaved move into the future, they do not need to sever the ties but to develop a new relationship with the deceased. The relationship of the past remains a part of who they are today and thus cherished (Silverman, 2001). Widowers reported that their positive feelings improved over time, especially if they were dating (Richardson & Balaswamy, 2001).

## Death of a Child

After a child's death, parents experience many different feelings. Feelings of grief may be so intense that parents do not realize what is happening to them. They may take part in activities they never did prior to their child's death and find meaning in the loss through these actions. Reilly-Smorawski et al. (2002) reported the parents' "life narratives become punctuated by their baby's death and that other experiences come to be understood as having occurred before or after this pivotal event" (p.31). In a study conducted by Wheeler (2001), 176 bereaved parents were polled. Questionnaire returns indicated that the most frequently mentioned responses were numbness and disbelief, with the most frequently mentioned initial emotional responses as anger, bitterness, pain, fear, and guilt. Parents who reported being preoccupied with their child worried whether their child suffered and wanted to protect and hold their child. Current responses reported were continued questioning about why it happened, acceptance, and also an inability to accept the death. The study found that parents attempted to find meaning in their lives as well as making meaning of the death through contact with people and helping others.

As nurses provide support to those who grieve, they can think about what the death means to this person at this point in their life. As days, months, and years pass, the meaning of the experience will change. After 3 years, grieving mothers reported experiencing personal growth and felt as though they had more compassion, more tolerance, and more forgiveness as a result of their grief. (Hogan, Greenfield, & Schmidt, 2001).

Nurses can recommend support groups for grieving parents in order for them to share their life narrative. Many bereaved parents have found comfort in attending a Compassionate Friends support group, which is a mutual assistance self-help organization offering friendship and understanding to bereaved parents after the death of a child. Siblings are also invited to attend these groups.

Nurses are also part of a support network that helps parents accept the reality of the loss. A bereaved mother may be better able to accept the reality that her child has died when she is encouraged to hold, name, and baptize her dead newborn, then is given the opportunity to keep the newborn's significant mementos (Engler & Lasker, 2000). The staff becomes instrumental in helping the mother cope with the loss. For example, after the death of an infant, the NICU staff can offer a bereavement packet that includes photos, footprints, a memory certificate, and if desired by the family, visits by the chaplain or home clergy (Reilly-Smorawski et al., 2002). These bereavement packets become significant mementos to grieving parents. In acknowledging the baby's life and death, this kind of sensitivity will help the parents.

When a baby dies, parents are dealing with the loss of their child. They have dreamed of bringing home a healthy infant. When a child is born with a disability, the parents also mourn the loss of their dream of the healthy child. If that child dies, they mourn the death of a disabled child. "Regardless of severity of the impairment, every father described the special memories and joys inherent to his child's spirit or personality" (Wood & Milo, 2000, pg. 651). Whether parents are describing the brief memories of their child or blaming themselves,

nurses should reassure them, provide comfort, and address their sense of responsibility.

A grieving mother often repeatedly asks, "Why did it happen? Did I cause it?" As the nurse attempts to answer unanswerable questions, it helps to focus on the need to allow the mother to ask the questions and not on needing to have answers. Sometimes, no matter what is said, the grieving person may continue to ask questions. Even many years after a child's death, parents feel extreme passion in not letting go of their deceased children. Despite the passage of time, one 85-year-old mother acknowledged that she still felt guilty that her infant child died (Riches & Dawson, 2002). After a child's death, the nurse can listen to parents share their concerns and their sense of responsibility. Listening to parents express their culpability is an important step in their trying to answer questions that sometimes have no answers. Though it may be distressing, communicating these concerns will help them cope with the loss.

A bereaved mother said,

It's a continual process, and people who say it ends after whatever (two years or a year) or that after the first year you should be okay, that's crazy! It's not a true adage. Time does change you and you can adapt to change, but for me it doesn't heal the scar that's left. Even after twenty years, you still remember, it still hurts, and no matter what people tell you, this will never go away (Eakes, Burke, & Hainsworth, 1999, p 177).

One of the most devastating experiences for adults is the death of their child. After 31 months, one grieving mother said, "Her death has changed my life profoundly and I feel like a completely different person. It's like a part of me died and a stronger part took its place" (Uren & Wastell 2002, p. 301). One of the most significant and consistent findings of recent studies is that parents mourn the death of their child and attempt to find meaning in the loss. A 31-year-old bereaved father of a premature son said, "I look forward to someday seeing his sweet little face in heaven" (Gamino, Hogan, & Sewell, 2002, p. 807).

There is stress and strain on marital relationships after the death of a child. Kastenbaum (1999) discussed common effects on the marital relationships. The first effect is serious repercussions for the bereaved couple's sexuality, from no intimacy to increased need for physical contact. Another common effect is feeling more irritable, being angry at each other, and blaming one another. A third common effect on marital relationships is communication breakdown, where the husband and wife move into their grief and away from one another. The last common effect is the shutdown of self-disclosure of emotional exchange through denial or intellectualization of feelings, a pattern at times identified as the conspiracy of silence.

### Perinatal Loss

For those who work with the bereaved, perinatal loss includes losses from the time of conception though the first 28 days of life (Rybarik, 2000). There are 6.9 infant deaths per 1,000 live births (Arias & Smith, 2003). The leading cause of infant mortality is congenital malformation (see Table 7-1). Many bereaved parents are young and have not experienced someone close to them dying. They have expected their baby to survive, and the sudden loss causes an empty space in their lives. Grout and Romanoff (2000) found that grieving parents spoke about the empty space they felt right after their loss and that this empty space violated their expectations. After a perinatal loss, mothers continued to feel connected and close to their babies, and this continued relationship was not related to the time of birth that since past (Uren & Wastell, 2002).

> **Personal Insight**
> *What is your opinion about having a funeral for a stillborn child?*

Grout and Romanoff (2000) found that during early bereavement, some of the parents created rituals to do by themselves or as a family. Whether

| TABLE 7-1: INFANT DEATHS AND INFANT MORTALITY | |
| --- | --- |
| Certain infectious and parasitic diseases | 576 |
| Certain intestinal infectious diseases | 10 |
| Diarrhea and gastroenteritis of infectious origin | 1 |
| Tuberculosis | 1 |
| Tetanus | - |
| Diphtheria | - |
| Whooping cough | 13 |
| Meningococcal infection | 18 |
| Septicemia | 334 |
| Congenital syphilis | 1 |
| Gonococcal infection | - |
| Viral diseases | 114 |
| All causes | 27,798 |

*Source:* Arias, E. & Smith, B.L. (2003). *Death: Preliminary data for 2001.* National Vital Statistics Reports, 51(5), March 14, 2003.

planting a rose bush or tree, lighting memorial candles, looking at photo albums, or keeping a journal, parents found comfort in ritualization. The rituals are a way of keeping connected to the deceased child; they also help the griever have a sense of control over the situation. The helpful attributes found in women who experienced perinatal loss were a sense of personal control and active orientation. After the loss of a fetus or infant, many women felt that the loss in their life was inevitable and that it was an experience of growth. In the growth experience, they actively oriented themselves by seeking and using support as they attempted to make sense out of the death of their fetus or infant. (Lang, Goulet, Aita, Giguere, Lamarre, & Perreault, 2001). Nurses are in a position to provide support to grieving adult mothers as well as adolescent mothers.

Wheeler and Austin (2000) studied the mourning patterns of six bereaved adolescent mothers aged 15 to 17 who lost an infant to stillbirth or neonatal death. These mothers reported several feelings similar to those of older bereaved mothers: anxiety, searching, longing, and going crazy. The authors found four of the six mothers made poor decisions regarding dating and sex after the death. It was difficult for the bereaved adolescent mothers to return to life as it was before the loss. All the mothers reported their relationships with their friends had changed. Their peers were not mature enough or perhaps had not enough experience in grief to provide bereavement support. None of the mothers were given educational or emotional support from the hospital after the death. However, nurses can offer both educational as well as emotional support to these mothers to help them cope. Welch and Bergen (1999-2000) found that adolescent mothers had difficulty with separation issues and peer relationships. By understanding the special needs of adolescent mothers, nurses can be effective in providing care during the loss experience.

## Traumatic Loss

Traumatic losses occur through events that happen beyond the normal range of experience. Some causes are homicide, disaster, car crashes, multiple losses, public tragedy, and suicide. Common responses are shattered assumptions about the world, flashbacks, fear and anger, survivor guilt, attempts to find meaning, crying, and wailing. Let's begin this section by looking at homicide.

### Homicide

Homicide occurs when one person kills another person. It is recognized as a criminal act even if no body or weapon is found. In 2000, there were 16,765 homicides in the United States (Anderson, 2002). Most homicides are committed by individuals who know their victim. For example, many homicides are committed by current intimate partners or by previous boyfriends or spouses. Approximately one in three female homicide deaths are committed by an intimate partner, where only 5% of male homicide victims are killed by intimate partners (Paolozzi, Saltzman, Thompson, & Holmgreen, 2001).

In 2000, homicide was the fourth ranking cause of death for 10 to 14-year-olds and the second ranking cause of death for 15 to 19-year-olds (National Center for Health Statistics, 2002). If the child was taken to the hospital, very little was under the parent's control when they first arrived. The physicians and nurses were busy with patients, and the parents may have had to wait for information. Research on families after the violent death of a child or young adult by accident, homicide, or suicide indicates that the grief experienced by both parents may disrupt the cohesion and function of the family, which can lead to mental distress. (Lohan & Murphy, 2002). According to Wickie and Marwit (2000-2001),

> The parents of murdered children report more negative views of the benevolence of the world and confirms anecdotal discussions in the literature that parents of murdered children see people and events more negatively and that these negative views are a result of the special circumstances surrounding homicide, such as the act of murder itself, the additional trauma of investigations, prolonged judiciary proceedings, increased isolation, and intense anger at perpetrators (p. 110).

Parents whose children die suddenly tend to isolate themselves from society. Their tendency to withdraw is linked to factors common in parents whose child died in sudden traumatic ways, including feelings of guilt and self-blame about their child's death (Dyregrov, Nordanger, & Dyregrov, 2003).

Hatton (2003) found that less than one-fifth of respondents identified guilt or self-blame as a major difficulty for homicide survivors. This finding may be due to victims' rights advocates who have been helping homicide survivors cope with their loss. Respondents in this study reported severe emotional pain as the greatest difficulty. They also reported constantly searching for why the murder happened as well as rage and anger about the murder. After a sudden violent death, Rubel (1999d) suggests,

Mourning and recovery are more difficult because of the violent and sudden nature of their loss; therefore, professional assistance during these first few hours is essential as the survivors try to cope with the news of the death within the framework of their cultural and religious beliefs (p. 380).

Though violent death is a major public problem in the United States, there is no gold standard of bereavement services offered to family survivors to help them adjust (Murphy, 2000). Gamino, Sewell and Easterling (2000) found,

When focusing on personal growth as a positive outcome following bereavement, four factors emerged as correlates of better adjustment: ability to see some good resulting from the death, having a chance to say goodbye to the loved one, intrinsic spirituality, and spontaneous positive memories of the decedent (p. 638).

In a hospital setting, the nurse can provide immediate support to those bereaved by homicide by giving them the opportunity to be with their dead loved one and provide a place to share the experience while validating their loss.

## Disaster

A disaster can happen at any moment and can cause major loss of health, life, and property. Disasters such as earthquakes, tornados, and explosions may impact many people at one time, whether due to natural or human factors. Disasters also affect communities at local, national, or international levels.

The initial stage of a disaster is the impact. Disasters may or may not arise due to an intentional act, either anticipated or unexpected. Those affected include the dead, survivors, witnesses, first responders, bereaved relatives and friends, other responders, and local citizens. The time immediately after the disaster is when first responders attempt to save lives and property. After doing all that they can do, they then leave the disaster area. However, the impli-

cations of the disaster may last for some time, perhaps a lifetime. The impact of a disaster on an individual's functioning will depend on many factors.

Assumptions and Principles about Psychosocial Aspects of Disasters (Adachi et al., 2002) lists common factors that increase the risk of lasting problems.

a. Prior vulnerability to stress and loss

b. Deaths that are unexpected and untimely

c. Experiencing or witnessing horrific or terrifying events

d. Deaths attributable to human agency

e. Multiple losses and concurrent crises

f. Child whose parent dies in the disaster

g. Parents whose child dies in the disaster

h. Absence of or undue delay in the recovery of intact bodies of those killed in the disaster

(p. 458)

Following the September 11th terrorist attacks, the US Dept. of Health and Human Services (DHHS) offered grief and emotional response advice for children and adults. Resources for grief counseling and mental health services after a disaster are included (see Figure 7-2).

## Accidents

An accident can happen anywhere. In American homes, there is a fatal injury every 16 minutes and a disabling injury every 4 seconds (National Safety Council, 2003). An accident is an unexpected happening that occurs by chance or arises from unknown causes where there is a loss, bodily injury, or property damage. Such unfortunate events can result from carelessness, unawareness, ignorance, or a combination of causes. As a result of unintentional injuries, each year more than 90,000 people die in the U.S. Common types of accidents include falls; motor vehicle crashes; solid, liquid, gas, or vapor poisoning; drowning; firearms; and suffocation. In 2001, hundreds of infants died by accidents (see Table 7-2).

## FIGURE 7-2: GRIEF AND EMOTIONAL RESPONSE ADVICE

Resources for grief counseling and mental health services following the Sept. 11th terrorist acts in New York, Washington, D.C., and Somerset County, Pa., are available from the U.S. Department of Health and Human Services.

"The horror of these events is palpable to all of us, and they will have near-term and long-term effects," said HHS Secretary Tommy G. Thompson. "While HHS is helping the directly affected areas plan for concentrated long-term mental health services, it is also important to realize that all Americans have been impacted by the pictures and the reality of this destruction, and we will all need to work through this horror. We need to talk with our children, we need to support one another, and many adults may feel overwhelmed by these events. HHS wants to share the resources to confront and live through these traumatic events."

Advice for parents and children, rescue workers, and for all others nationwide for coping with emotional stress is available on the HHS website: ***TIPS FOR TALKING ABOUT DISASTERS***: http://www.mentalhealth.org/cmhs/EmergencyServices/after.htm

In addition, those needing personal guidance can call the toll-free hotline maintained by HHS' Substance Abuse and Mental Health Administration (SAMHSA) for counseling and referral to local resources nationwide: **1-800-789-2647 (TDD: 301-443-9006).**

In his visit to New York City Sept. 13, Gov. George Pataki, Mayor Rudolph Giuliani and New York health officials told Secretary Thompson that long-term planning and support for mental health services would be among the highest priority long-term needs for the city. SAMHSA officials traveled to New York that day to help advise and assist the city in planning for the long-term need, with financial and technical help from HHS. In addition, grant assistance for mental health relief was included in the first funding released by HHS Sept. 13 to address consequences of the disasters.

**General advice includes:**

**For children:** Answer questions honestly, but without dwelling on frightening details—but don't be afraid to admit you can't answer everything. Encourage expression of feelings and give opportunities to talk. Acknowledge your own feelings. Try to maintain normal routines, while also reducing sources of tension where possible. For younger children especially, cuddling as well as verbal support may be important. Teens especially may need to understand that hateful language and striking back can cause harm rather than help.

**For reassuring affected adults:** Important to acknowledge that reactions of grief and fear are normal—fear, irritability, crying, confusion. Important to know "it's not your fault, you did the best you could." Acknowledge that things may never be the same, but they will get better. Things to AVOID saying: "It could have been worse. You can always get another [pet/car/house/etc.]. It's best if you just stay busy. You need to get on with your life. I know just how you feel."

*Source*: United States Department of Health and Human Services. (2001). Grief and emotional response advice. HHS Press Office. http://www.hhs.gov/news/press/2001pres/20010915.html

The class of an accident is established by the location where it occurs, such as motor vehicle accidents, work-related accidents, injuries at home, and accidents in public. For example, nearly 20,000 Americans died of drug-induced causes in 2000, and another 20,000 died of alcohol-related causes (Anderson, 2002). Falls took the lives of 9,000 people, four out of five of them over the age of 65 (National Safety Council, 2003). Another type of accident is medical accidents, where an avoidable personal injury is caused by a medical treatment or failure to diagnose.

Accidents, homicides, and suicides account for 80% of all deaths among youth and young adults in

| TABLE 7-2: INFANT ACCIDENTAL DEATH | |
|---|---|
| Falls | 23 |
| Accidental discharge of firearms | - |
| Accidental drowning and submersion | 69 |
| Accidental suffocation and strangulation in bed | 347 |
| Other accidental suffocation and strangulation | 151 |
| Accidental inhalation and ingestion of food or other objects causing obstruction of respiratory tract | 56 |
| Accidents caused by exposure to smoke, fire and flames | 52 |
| Accidental poisoning and to noxious substances | 15 |
| Other and unspecified accidents | 59 |

*Source:* Arias, E. & Smith, B.L. (2003). Deaths: Preliminary data for 2001. *National Vital Statistics Reports, 51*(5), March 14, 2003.

the US (US. Bureau of the Census, 1999). Motor vehicle crashes are the leading cause of death for people age 1 to 33, and the age groups most affected by these crashes are 15-24 and 75+ (National Safety Council, 2003). After the sudden death of a child, parents will feel intense emotional reactions (such as guilt, separation, difficult accepting the death, and helplessness). When a death occurs due to a car crash, survivors often experience anger. Their anger is often manifested as rage if the death was caused by the negligence of a drunken driver (Rubel, 1999d). When a child is killed in a traffic accident, parents grieve for several years. After the traumatic loss of their child, parents have reported that they need detailed information given to them, especially medical information related to the death; a reconstruction of what happened; compassionate caregivers; and an opportunity to spend time alone with the child, to hold the child and say goodbye (Spooren, Henderich, & Jannes, 2000). In their study of parents whose children died in a traffic accident, though the majority of parents indicated that support was available, half of the parents reported being unsatisfied with the services they received after the loss, the medical interventions, the time and space they were allowed to be with their child, and the information about the circumstances of their child's death.

Though there was no correlation between the age of the child killed and parental bereavement problems, parents do feel psychological suffering for many years after the death. Parents reported the need:

1. for detailed information; including medical information related to the death,

2. to make a reconstruction of what happened,

3. for a friendly and compassionate attitude of the caretakers,

4. to spend some time alone with the child, to be able to hold their child and to say goodbye

(Spooren, Henderich, & Jannes, 2000, p. 180).

The National Center for Injury Prevention and Control (NCIPC) reports that two out of five deaths among U.S. teens are the resut of a motor vehicle crash (NCIPC, 2004). Sudden, unexpected death seems to create a debilitating shock in the bereaved, which may extend the grief response and create extreme physical and emotional trauma (Straub & Roberts, 2001). Survivors cannot be shielded from the reality of death in a car crash. Nurses can provide grief support by identifying the tasks that the bereaved need to do, finding out what the survivors need, and identifying ways for them to help themselves.

**Multiple Deaths**

Adults may experience anxiety, anger, and depression after multiple deaths. There is a cumulative impact of these deaths on the survivor's ability to mourn. Those in the gay community have lost many of their friends to AIDS. A total of 14,478 people died from HIV/AIDS in 2000 (NCHS, 2002). Year after year the bereaved attend funerals and feel saddened by the multiple losses. Those who are HIV-positive or who have AIDS face their own mortality each time another friend dies. HIV ranks 5th among the leading causes of death for all persons between the ages of 35 and 44, but 2nd among Hispanic males of that age group and 1st among African-American males of that age (NCHS, 2002).

The grieving individual may find it difficult to cope when bereaved by two or more significant deaths. Becoming pessimistic and socially withdrawing are common responses while fearing additional losses. By socially withdrawing from family and friends, and not attempting to meet someone new, there is less risk of experiencing another loss. However, there is greater risk of anger, which can be especially intense after the death of a young person. When several young people are killed in an accident at the same time, or when a young person completes suicide and later another student in that family or community also completes suicide, the mourners attempt to cope with being separated from the deceased. If the death was violent, separation distress symptoms, such as yearning, are more common than for those whose relatives experienced an accidental death (Prigerson et al., 1997).

A total of 28,663 people died from firearms in 2000 (NCHS, 2003b). Among those aged 19 and under, the number of firearm deaths decreased by more than 10 percent compared with 1999 (NCHS, 2003b). When several people are killed, especially by gunshot, the multiple deaths are more difficult to accept and understand. As the bereaved grieve, intrusive thoughts of the deceased come to mind. Thoughts include the pain the person may have experienced and the fear felt moments before dying. Individuals may find intrusive thoughts very disturbing. A recent study found that intrusive memories were more common in those bereaved by suicide and accidents than parents bereaved by SIDS, who showed significantly fewer problems (Dyregrov, Nordanger, & Dyregrov, 2003).

---

*Personal Insight*

*Have you experienced multiple losses in your life? If so, have you experienced intrusive thoughts? What were the thoughts and how did you cope with them?*

---

## Public Tragedy

Doka (2003) notes factors that influence the public perception of tragedy. The larger the scope of the tragedy, the more likely the tragedy will be considered public. If we identify with the victim or victims and if they have greater social value because of their status, the death will be perceived as a public tragedy. Other factors include the consequences of the death and the duration, especially if the tragedy happened suddenly. On September 11, 2001, thousands of individuals died from terrorism when planes crashed in New York City, Virginia, and Pennsylvania (Arias & Smith, 2003).

The natural-to-human continuum can influence perception, as individuals struggle with whether the tragedy was due to a natural act such as a hurricane or a human act, such as terrorism. What caused the public tragedy will have a direct bearing on how people feel about it. In a natural public tragedy, individuals may be angry toward God. However, in a human caused tragedy, the anger will be toward the person that caused the death. The degree of intentionality can also influence the public's perception of the tragedy. If it was a random act, the public may perceive the event as one that could have happened to them. If the public perceives the tragedy as intentional, they will assign blame. Though assigning blame will not make the public any safer, it will give them an illusion of safety. At least they have someone to blame as they attempt to react to the tragedy. Expectedness and preventability also influence public perception of tragedy as well as the greater perception of suffering. Greater perception of suffering involves whether the victims died instantly, and how much the victims suffered before dying. This perception of suffering will affect the way the public mourns the deaths.

The death of Princess Diana is another public tragedy that affected individuals from around the world who mourned her loss. Bull, Clark, and Duszynski (2002-2003), found that the responses of those seeking assistance after Diana's death wanted to talk at length about her death, resurfacing grief issues, expressing sorrow. Nurses may be called upon in public tragedies. The authors made the following suggestions to assist in future occurrences of community-wide-grief.

- Organizations should have distinct guidelines detailing appropriate strategies to deal with increased requests for assistance and support during such occurrences of grief.

- Organizations should ensure adequate numbers of support workers/staff are available, even if this requires utilizing "reserve" volunteers.

- Support staff should have access to their own support meetings and be able to implement additional debriefing sessions.

- Literature concerning grief and relevant support services should be available at large gatherings such as memorial services.

- Literature should detail elements of grief and other relevant issues, such as resurfacing of previous losses, and community members should be reassured their reactions to such devastating circumstances are normal.

- Such literature and information should be accessible in the print media, on television, and on radio.

- Hotlines should also be established to disseminate information as well as to advise people on more comprehensive paths of assistance.

- Large-scale services by religious and other group should be offered as another option for those wishing to express their grief.

- The media should be alerted to ways of sensitively and responsibly covering

tragedies, in recognition of the potential impact of media coverage on vulnerable grievers

(p. 44).

The public perception of Diana's tragic death was influenced by the media that became the eyes and ears for those around the world seeking information about the public tragedy. Mourners after Diana's death were consuming all available media coverage (Bull et al., 2002-2003).

> *Personal Insight*
> *Describe a public tragedy that happened in your lifetime. What emotions did you experience during and afterwards? Did the media coverage affect your response to the tragedy?*

# ELDERLY

## Encounters with Death and Bereavement

*Old age, terminal diseases, and life-ending traumas eventually become roads taking us to predictable endpoints* —Kessler, 1998, p.132

The emphasis thus far in this chapter has been on the issues faced by children, adolescents, and adults. This section focuses on the elderly: the "young old" (65-75), the "old" (75-85), and the oldest old (age 85+). Though humans' maximum potential life span is about 115 years, most American live about 76 years. The leading cause of death for those over the age of 65 is heart disease (Table 7-3). The longer a person lives, the more losses they experience in life. In the nineteenth century, there were very few grandparents in America, as individuals did not live long enough to see their grandchildren. Today, grandparents may lives miles away or live in the same home as their grandchildren. Whether they see their grandchildren remotely or share a much-involved relationship, they grieve the loss when the child dies. For those grandparents who take an active role in the care of their grandchildren, the grief response may

## TABLE 7-3: TEN LEADING CAUSES OF DEATH IN AMERICANS 65 AND OVER

| | |
|---|---|
| All causes | 1,801,303 |
| 1. Diseases of heart | 583,773 |
| 2. Malignant neoplasms | 389,657 |
| 3. Cerebrovascular diseases | 144,626 |
| 4. Chronic lower respiratory diseases | 107,787 |
| 5. Influenza and pneumonia | 55,668 |
| 6. Diabetes mellitus | 53,743 |
| 7 Alzheimer's disease | 53,078 |
| 8. Nephritis, nephritic syndrome and nephrosis | 33,260 |
| 9. Accidents (unintentional injuries) | 32,214 |
| Motor vehicle accidents | 7,166 |
| All other accidents | 25,048 |
| 10. Septicemia | 25,420 |
| All other cause (residual) | 322,077 |

*Source:* Arias, E. & Smith, B.L. (2003). Deaths: Preliminary data for 2001. *National Vital Statistics Reports, 51*(5), March 14, 2003.

be similar to that of the parents of the child. No matter what the bond, whether remote or extremely involved, grandparents will experience grief of the death of a grandchild.

An elderly person's grief response could include appetite changes, sleep disturbances, crying, anger, sadness, guilt, and helplessness. Grandparents experience a double grief, where they grieve for the loss of their grandchild and they grieve for their own children's pain of loss. As they see their child grieving, they may attempt to be strong in order to provide support. A nurse can encourage the grieving grandparent to express that grief openly in front of their children. Sharing their grief with their children will give the entire family an opportunity to talk with and listen to each other during this time. Grandparents should support and comfort those they love without losing sight of their own needs.

Grandparents attempting to adjust to their lives without their grandchild find support in talking with friends, neighbors, and family about the grandchild's death. They will mourn the loss of the child as well as mourn the loss of what the child was to become. They have probably assumed they would watch the child grow and carry on their name, so when the child dies, those dreams are shattered. Whether grandparents find comfort in talking about their grandchild, writing a letter to their grandchild, or keeping something that belonged to the grandchild, they feel the need to provide comfort to their own children. Doing so will help them cope with whatever they are feeling, especially if they are experiencing guilt. Most grandparents believe they will not outlive their grandchildren. When the grandchild dies, they may say, "It should have been me!" Talking with their children about their feelings will provide support and comfort.

Lund and Caserta (2002) point out,

Loneliness and problems associated with managing the tasks of daily living are two of the most common and difficult adjustments for older adults. These problems are even more difficult for the spousally bereaved because the daily lives of spouses are so closely connected. In later life, especially, spouses frequently become dependent on each other for conversation, love, and sharing of tasks. Loneliness is problematic because it involves missing, sadness, and a void that does not go away simply by being with or among other people (p. 211).

With this in mind, health professionals can recommend support groups for the bereaved, not only as a place to share their loss but also as a place to come together and socialize with others in similar situations. Often after a bereavement support group ends, several of the elderly members will exchange telephone numbers or meet for coffee before going home. They continue to talk about the relationships they shared with those that have died and their history of loss.

Very old bereaved persons place the death of their friends in the context of their life course and history of loss, with a profound sense of survivorship due to their outliving the significant people in their life (de Vries, Blieszner, & Blando, 2002).

One woman commented that she missed "not being necessary to anyone." One man, describing the circumstances following the death of his friend, said: "His family didn't seem to care much about him in his life. After his accident, they all came out to the coast, formed a sort of human shield around him denying us access to him or even knowledge about his condition. They swept through the house taking his belongings and left us with nothing — not even a chance to speak at the funeral (p. 235).

## Patterns of Adjustment

Adults adjust to aging and adjust to the reality that one day they will die. Aging is a life-long process that begins at conception; it is simply the process of growing older. As we age, adults may encounter all types of losses and accept their death is a part of life. Kelly (2001) maintains that acceptance includes:

a) the universality of loss and gain,

b) the natural cycle of life and death,

c) anger as a natural response to loss, and

d) grief as a normal process.

As adults adjust to the realities of their mortality, they realize that everyone will die and that it is a natural part of life. Some adults may be more anxious in that adjustment than others. DePaola, Griffin, Young, & Neimeyer (2003) found that elderly African-Americans were more anxious in regard to fear of the unknown, fear of consciousness when dead, and fear for the body after they died than were elderly caucasians. Elderly caucasians

reported higher levels of death anxiety on the fear of dying process than did elderly African-Americans. As men and women age and accept that death is a natural part of life, they are faced with issues of where they will spend the last days of their life. Elderly caucasians may experience greater death anxiety than African-Americans because most whites die in hospitals and nursing homes where they are isolated from family. Many of these elderly caucasians die in pain. Fear of a prolonged and painful dying is particularly evident among institutionalized older adults, which can be rationally supported and may perhaps give reasons for Caucasian families to be interested in palliative care interventions at the end of life (DePaola et al., 2003).

## Personal Control and Independence

Those who are 65 years of age and older want, as they grow older, personal control and independence to be maintained as they take part in decisions about their lives. Health care professionals can reassure them that their life is worth living. Their lives should not be devalued because they are elderly. When the elderly are faced with life-threatening illness and dying, they should participate in decisions regarding their care. As the highest rate of suicide is among the elderly, we must acknowledge their depression and help them maintain control.

# SUMMARY

This chapter has examined life span issues. Children's and adolescents encounters with death and bereavement were examined. Loss is experienced through an entire lifespan beginning in childhood. Silverman, Nickman, and Worden's five categories that reflect a child's efforts to maintain a connection to their deceased parent were examined. Within this chapter, children's understandings of death were noted. Though infants and toddlers may perceive that adults are sad or distraught, children this young have no real understanding of the meaning of death. The death perceptions of children between the ages of 2 and 4, 3 and 5, and 5 and 7 were examined. The aspects of children's understanding of death were noted, with most children understanding non-functionality, irreversibility, universality, causality, and personal mortality by about 10 years of age.

Within this chapter, the need to identify and assess the bereaved child was emphasized. The common emotional reactions, mental reactions, physical reactions, and behavioral reactions of grief were noted. Interventions with bereaved children and how they grieve in a family context were detailed. Children's tasks in coping with loss and grief and the significance of linking objects were noted.

This chapter also examined the ways adolescents understand death and common characteristics of grieving adolescents at different ages. Early adolescence (roughly ages 10 to 14) was discussed. Some of the changes facing middle adolescents (roughly age 15 to 16) and late adolescents (roughly ages 17 to 19) were noted. This chapter discussed interventions with bereaved adolescents. Also, ways nurses can notify adolescents that their loved one has died were explored. Suggestions for assisting adolescents who are coping with death and bereavement were offered.

The next part of this chapter explored adults view of their childhood bereavement. Experiences and encounters with death and bereavement and the unique grief of those who experience the death of a parent were discussed. Several of the ways widows remain emotionally and spiritually attached to the deceased were noted. Ways a nurse can address practical matters and offer advice and referrals were also discussed. The intense feelings of parents after the death of their child were then examined. Perinatal loss is a painful experience. Some of the rituals parents created as a way of keeping connected to the deceased child to help them have a sense of control over the situation were noted.

Near the end of this chapter, traumatic losses such as homicide and accidents were discussed.

Accidents in the home, falls, motor vehicle crashes, poisoning, drowning, firearms, suffocation, and medical accidents were listed. The intense emotional reactions of parents after the sudden death of their child, the significance of services received after the loss, and what the parent's needed immediately after the death were noted. Motor vehicle death rates and how sudden, unexpected death seems to create a debilitating shock in the bereaved was examined. Multiple deaths and the cumulative impact of these deaths on the survivor's ability to mourn were noted. References were made to those in the gay community as they have lost friends and partners to AIDS. Also, factors that influence the public after a public tragedy were identified.

Elderly encounters with death and bereavement were identified. The grief response of grandparents and suggestions for coping were noted. Patterns of adjustment to loss as we age were also identified. Universality of loss and gain, the natural cycle of life and death, grief as a natural response to loss, and age as a normal process were explored. The chapter concluded by examining elderly personal control and independence.

# RESOURCES

## Life Span Issues on the Internet

Alliance of Grandparents, a Support in Tragedy
　　www.agast.org

American Academy of Experts in Traumatic Stress
　　www.aaets.org

American Red Cross
　　www.redcross.org

The Dougy Center, GreivingChild.org
　　www.dougy.org

Grief Support for Children and Adolescents
　　www.funeralplan.com/griefsupport/
　　okay1.html

International Critical Incident Stress Foundation
　　www.icisf.org

Living with Grief: Children, Adolescents and Loss
www.hospicefoundation.org/lwg.htm

National Organization of Parents of Murdered
Children, Inc.
www.pomc.org

Office for Victims of Crime, US Dept. of Justice
www.ojp.usdoj.gov/ovc/

SHARE Pregnancy and Infant Loss Support
www.nationalshareoffice.com

receiving

# CHAPTER 7
### Questions 66-76

66. Children begin to understand the finality of death by the age of

a. 1-5 years.

b. 5-9 years.

c. 9-13 years.

d. 13-17 years.

67. The understanding that all life-sustaining functions cease with death is

a. non-functionality.

b. irreversibility.

c. universality.

d. personal mortality.

68. The understanding of personal mortality includes knowing that

a. death is final, and once dead, a person cannot become alive again.

b. all life-sustaining functions cease with death.

c. not only that all living things die but that "I will die."

d. philosophy aids in looking at what causes death.

69. One effective intervention with bereaved children is to

a. hold and rock them.

b. help them throw away or donate items that once belonged to their loved one.

c. keep them busy.

d. encourage them to move on.

70. A child's task in coping with loss and grief is to

a. understand and begin to let go of the bond shared with the deceased.

b. commemorate the death of the person.

c. learn to forget the pain of loss and move on with life.

d. identify, validate, and express in constructive ways their strong reactions to the loss.

71. When helping bereaved adolescents, adults should

a. identify previous losses and how they grieved in the past.

b. attempt to keep information secret to protect them.

c. not allow them to be with the dying person to protect them.

d. not allow them to attend the funeral or partake in any funeral planning.

72. According to Flemming and Balmer, death impacts the lives of adolescents as seen in

a. friendships and school performance.

b. school performance and self-esteem.

c. family relationships and school performance.

d. self-esteem and friendships.

73. In a study conducted by Wheeler, two most frequently mentioned responses found in parents after the death of their child are

    a. numbness and disbelief.

    b. sadness and acceptance.

    c. numbness and rage.

    d. shame and anger.

74. A common effect on the marital relationship after the death of a child is

    a. serious repercussions for the bereaved couple's sexuality, from no intimacy to increased need for physical contact.

    b. feeling less irritable, not being angry at each other, and not blaming one another.

    c. communication enhancement, where the husband and wife move away from their grief and toward one another.

    d. the revival of self-disclosure of emotional exchange through acceptance of feelings.

75. A significant and consistent finding in parents after the death of their child is

    a. mourning the death of their child and having other children.

    b. reading books on child loss and setting up a memorial in the name of their child.

    c. mourning the death of their child and attempting to find meaning in the loss.

    d. reading books on child loss and caring for their other children.

76. Two of the most common and difficult adjustments for grieving older adults are

    a. fear and no longer being dependent on someone.

    b. not being able to have a conversation and sleeping with someone.

    c. loneliness and problems associated with managing the tasks of daily living.

    d. being with or among other people and eating healthy food.

# CHAPTER 8

# ROLE OF SOCIAL SUPPORT IN BEREAVEMENT

## CHAPTER OBJECTIVE

After completing this chapter, the reader will be able to identify various means of bereavement support.

## LEARNING OBJECTIVES

After studying this chapter, the reader will be able to

1. specify ways bereavement support groups and bereavement counseling provides support to the bereaved.

2. identify common problems found in bereavement support groups.

3. differentiate between Internet bereavement support and psycho-educational workshops.

## INTERVENTIONS

### Bereavement Counseling

As the bereaved reach out for support, they have several options. One such option is meeting with a bereavement or grief counselor. Grief counseling provides support to those who have experienced a loss. The term counseling, as used in this book, encompasses the professional forms of helping those who are bereaved.

Bereavement counselors developed specialized skills through appropriate training and experience.

Although the task of helping grieving family members seems daunting, providing assistance during this difficult time will help the family accept the finality of death and address any problems and complications. Fauri, Ettner, and Kovacs (2000) note that bereavement services help reduce the immediate physical and emotional distress of those who mourn. By educating the bereaved about the grief process and offering information about support networks in their community, those who grieve are given a powerful tool to heal. Clinicians assist grieving widowers by giving them a chance to speak about their wives' deaths and the circumstances surrounding their loss (Richardson & Balaswamy, 2001). The sorrow one feels over the loss of a loved one can last a lifetime. Chronic sorrow is triggered by events and moments in life. As time moves on, periods of happiness blend into moments of sadness.

Eakes, Burke, and Hainsworth (1999) studied individuals who experienced chronic sorrow and asked them what they believed was helpful as they revisited their grief. Those who experienced the death of a significant other made two recommendations to health care professionals who help those experiencing chronic sorrow. One helpful role was being an empathetic presence by listening and being supportive as they focused on feelings and the uniqueness of the griever. The second helpful role was one of being a caring professional. Those who offer bereavement counseling should take into consideration what the bereaved may be experiencing.

They will express their grief and appreciate a counselor who allows them to feel comfortable doing so.

By asking the bereaved certain questions, the nurse can assess if they are in need of bereavement counseling. It is not the role of nurses to provide bereavement counseling. The nurse is not always in a position to provide this counseling. Intervention by the nurse helps when we show concern, allow survivors them to view the body, and give them an opportunity to call their clergy or other family members. Due to time constraints, it is not always possible for nurses to explore issues of the relationship, the type of loss, and the support system in place. However, if any of the following recommended key questions could be asked of the bereaved, it would provide insight into their bereavement needs. Raphael, Middleton, Martinek, and Misso (1997) recommend the following key questions when assessing and planning care of the bereaved to see if they are vulnerable and in need of bereavement counseling.

- Can you tell me about him/her?

- Can you tell me about the death, how he/she died?

- Can you tell me about how others have responded to you since — what they said and did, what it meant to you?

- Can you tell me about the other things that have happened to you, or are happening now, that are making things harder for you as well?

- Can you tell me about yourself, as a person, and your life before all this happened — how has it been, and what sorts of things have you had to face in the past?

- Can you tell me about the family — how this has affected the family as a whole, and what you feel it has meant for each person?

(p. 429).

Depending upon the responses, the nurse can see if there are any particular difficulties the individual is facing and offer support. Support can be found in various forms of grief counseling.

Parkes (1980) outlines three basic types of grief counseling.

1. Professional services by trained doctors, nurses, psychologists, or social workers who provide support to a person who has sustained a significant loss.

2. Services in which volunteers are selected, trained, and supported by professionals

3. Self-help groups in which bereaved people offer help to other bereaved people, with or without the support of professionals.

After the death of a loved one, the bereaved begin a self-reflective process that helps them cope. They can choose any of the three basic types of grief counseling or explore ways on their own that help them process their grief. By using the self-reflective process of journaling and conversation with oneself, a better self-awareness may arise (Danforth & Glass, 2001). Some of the topics of reflections include:

a) expressions of grief,

b) identity in the married relationship,

c) new relationships,

d) affirmation,

e) successful experiences,

f) sources of personal strength,

g) assumptions about life, and

h decision-making avenues of interests.

# BEREAVEMENT SUPPORT GROUPS

Stylianos and Vachon (1997) addressed social support in bereavement support groups. The authors maintain that additional social support can benefit the bereaved. Support can initially be found in the person's pre-existing social network. At the outset, the bereaved can primarily be supported by family and friends, bereavement professionals, or a member of a self-help support group. However, the authors note that at a later point during their bereavement, friends can become essential in providing support and this support can be found in a self-help program. The self-help program might be beneficial as the group members provide help to one another during their grief.

Fauri et al. (2000) point out the significance of providing help to the family immediately following their loss, as it helps preserve the family and their well-being. An important intervention that the nurse can recommend is a bereavement support group. These groups can help those who have experienced unsupportive social interaction after the loss of their loved one. Ingram, Jones, and Smith (2001) maintain that if professionals fail to address the "unhelpful, unsupportive, or distressing responses that a bereavement client may have received from other people concerning his or her experience of loss, they may fail to identify an important part of the client's bereavement experience" (p. 305).

Support groups are places of empathy, acceptance, safety, and growth. The group becomes a place where grieving individuals can share their grief and come to realize that what they are feeling is normal. A widow of 15 months stated, "I have pretty much gotten over the acute pain of my husband's death but still feel that I need to go back to my support group from time to time so I can still talk about him" (Ott & Lueger, 2002, p. 404).

Grief is facilitated in support groups in a variety of ways.

- Discussing the changes in one's life since the death.

- Remembering and sharing the memories with those who have experienced similar losses.

- Normalizing feelings.

- Telling and retelling one's story.

- Sharing pictures and objects that once belonged

to the deceased.

- Providing information to the bereaved on the grief process.

- Exploring spiritual activities that bring comfort.

- Encouraging forgiveness.

Picton, Cooper, Close, and Tobin (2001) found that people join bereavement support groups when they felt it was the right time, whether immediately after the death, weeks, months, or even years later, when they wanted to be with and share with others who have experienced similar losses. Many participants reported feelings of isolation, hopelessness, depression, and suicide ideation, particularly those whose loss was recent. Based on these feelings, they believed they needed professional help and that the group would provide such a forum to discuss their feelings. Murphy, Clark-Johnson, and Lohan (2003) studied 138 grieving parents after the violent death of their child. The authors found that parents who went to bereavement support groups were 4 times more likely to find meaning in their child's death than parents who did not attend the groups 5 years postdeath. Nearly everyone in a study by Geron, Ginzburg, and Solomon (2003) reported joining support groups to develop relationships with others in similar situations, to gain coping skills, and to make contact with experts in the field of bereavement.

To provide a healing forum to share their feelings, a professionally run bereavement support group must follow certain guidelines in order to be most effective. The facilitator runs the group and orients those present by providing information. This information can include time frame, group participation expectations, privacy issues, confidentiality, and group goals. A handout should be provided that includes information about the group and the qualifications of the facilitator.

A bereavement self-help group is a support group that offers mutual aid, it becomes a support system for the bereaved and run by the bereaved.

The facilitator is an individual who, in most cases, has experienced a death of someone close to them.

Lieberman (1997) maintains,

Regardless of the type of group, participants uniformly indicated that such groups provided an important source of "normalization" or "universalization" (the problem they bring to the group is often experienced as shameful and abhorrent; finding others with the same problem solving support (p.412).

Lieberman notes the benefits of self-help groups include the low cost and that the group is usually based in the community. Whether professionally run, facilitated by volunteers, or run by the bereaved themselves, bereavement groups help the bereaved address their reactions and any distress they may be experiencing. This is an essential aspect of bereavement services, which provide a forum for those who mourn to process the death.

Those who attend a bereavement support group may not wish to address their grief and bereavement issues. They may simply want information or socializing. Two types of groups meet these unique needs. The first type of support group is for those grievers who want to socialize. These men and women meet for bus trips, group walks on the boardwalk, meals at restaurants, and theatre performances. The aim of attending this type of support group is to be with other grievers and meet people. The bereaved may be lonely, and this type of group brings them together with others who share similar activities.

Another form of support is an informational type of support group. Those who attend this type of group want to learn ways to live their life in a more constructive way. After a spouse dies, making meals or filling out a tax return may be difficult tasks. Having guest speakers and experts at the group meeting to present on various topics related to the unique needs of those who mourn can assist the bereaved in making life adjustments (i.e. filling out a tax return, preparing a living wills, cooking).

# COMMON PROBLEMS IN BEREAVEMENT SUPPORT GROUPS

Bereavement support groups are valuable to those who want to share their story. However, there are common problems found in bereavement groups. Participants can become frustrated by the unending talker who dominates the conversation so often that others in the group are not given the opportunity to share their stories of loss. In this case, the facilitator should mention the purpose of the group and concentrate on the group as a place of coming together to share stories and pain of loss. Though it is a time of listening, if one member speaks for an extended period of time, others will not have the opportunity to speak.

A common problem found in bereavement support groups is the group member who takes the role of the liberator. The liberator attempts to rescue the group members from their pain of loss. The liberator will commonly use clichés to help group members with such statements as, "Everything will be okay." Unhelpful statements are not effective in helping group members cope with their grief. If the group facilitator is not trained to deal with the liberator, he or she will continue to say the wrong things and be ineffective in providing support.

Another problem with bereavement support groups is the member who takes on the role of captain. He or she attempts to run the ship, so to speak. The captain ignores the fact that a group facilitator is present and attempts to run things. If the group facilitator is untrained in dealing with this type of behavior, others in the group will wind up leaving as they sense the facilitator is not in control of the bereavement group.

One of the biggest problems in bereavement support groups is the way the facilitator deals with a crying member. When a member cries, he or she is expressing an emotion. It is not up to the group facilitator to stop the tears. Some facilitators quickly hand the bereaved a tissue. Though they mean well by handing the person a tissue, those facilitators are, in essence, telling the person to stop crying and dry their tears.

> ### Personal Insight
> *Think of a time when you were in a group situation where there was a problem staff member or patient. What would you do if you were responsible for that individual?*

Due to problems with support group members, grieving individuals may choose to stop attending meetings and choose to share their loss with grieving individuals on the Internet. Bereavement support groups are not limited to real time.

## INTERNET BEREAVEMENT SUPPORT

Online bereavement support groups and networks are open to worldwide membership. Message threads are posted on boards and relief from isolation is found. Though there is no actual leader or facilitator, each individual plays an integral role. The bereaved are finding self-help through mailing lists, listservs, and web sites that offer support 24 hours a day. For those who cannot drive to a support group or who are not comfortable sharing their grief in a group, they can find comfort and support in the privacy of their home. A study examining the link between support found through the Internet and healing has provided a notable finding. Rich (2000) found that after a perinatal loss, parents found support through Internet e-mail perinatal bereavement support groups. Bereaved parents also join perinatal bereavement support groups to meet with others who have experienced similar losses.

There are support groups and chat rooms for those patients who are living with a life-threatening illness. Caregivers can benefit from this on-line support, which helps them with feelings of isolation and alienation. Though Internet support groups provide patients with an opportunity to reach out to those with similar issues and concerns, home care nurses should speak with their patients about the risks involved. Patients and family members should not confuse information and suggestions from the lay group with a recognized professional's information, and they should not take the advice of the group over that of their physician, nurse, or primary provider. They should know not to offer personal information and that some people on the Internet may be offensive (Martin & Youngren, 2000).

One aim of creating a personal web site is to share one's story, reach out to others who share similar experiences, and learn their approach to healing. Madara (1999) maintains,

> Online groups and networks meet the needs of those who seek support, education and advocacy by offering:
>
> 1. social support,
> 2. practical information,
> 3. shared experiences,
> 4. positive role models,
> 5. helper therapy,
> 6. empowerment,
> 7. professional support,
> 8. advocacy efforts, and
> 9. accessibility
> (p.45).

## PSYCHO-EDUCATIONAL WORKSHOPS

Psycho-educational workshops offer the bereaved an opportunity to learn about death, dying, and bereavement. An overriding goal of psycho-educational workshops is to empower the participants by offering information that guides them in understanding the topic and how it relates to their experience. The presenter's goal in facilitating the workshop is to address the concerns and issues facing the group.

Psycho-educational workshops offer information, opportunities for understanding, and support. One such situation involves those who are affected by a death in the line of military duty. Each Memorial Day Weekend, friends and families come together at the Annual National Military Survivor Seminar in Washington, DC. For 3 days, workshops are offered from leading experts in the field of trauma and grief. These workshops are not limited to family and friends. Chaplains, ombudsmen, commanders, family support personnel, and others also attend to learn valuable information that will help those who seek their support. These workshops can include helping families cope with loss and financial planning among other topics related to death in the line of military duty.

Another psycho-educational workshop takes place each May during National Police Week in Washington, DC. The Concerns Of Police Survivors, Inc. (COPS) host the National Police Survivors' Conference for law enforcement survivors, co-workers, family, and friends. Some of the workshops are related to drunken driving incidents, heart attacks, natural causes, and suicides. These workshops educate and empower the survivors as they share their grief with others who have experienced similar types of losses.

# SUMMARY

This chapter reviewed the role of social support in bereavement. This chapter started with some of the interventions in bereavement counseling. Questions when assessing and planning care of the bereaved to see if they are vulnerable and in need of bereavement counseling were discussed. Three basic types of grief counseling and the self-reflective process of journaling and conversation with oneself to help cope with loss were noted.

In this chapter, bereavement support groups, where the bereaved want to be with and share with others who have experienced similar losses were examined. Differences were noted between professionally run groups, self-help groups, informational type groups, socialization bereavement support groups, and Internet support groups. Some of the problems that group facilitators can experience with certain members of any group were reviewed. The chapter concluded by highlighting psycho-educational workshops, which offer the bereaved an opportunity to learn about death, dying, and bereavement.

# RESOURCES

## Role of Social Support in Bereavement on the Internet

The American Academy of Bereavement
   http://www.bereavementacademy.org

The Compassionate Friends (TCF)
   www.compassionatefriends.org

National Center for Death Education
   http://www.mountida.edu/sp.cfm?pageid=307

RTS Bereavement Services
   (loss of an infant through miscarriage, stillbirth, or neonatal death)
   http://www.llu.edu/llumc/nursing/rts.htm

Bereaved Parents of the U.S.A.
   www.bereavedparentsusa.org

SHARE
   (early pregnancy loss, stillbirth or newborn death)
   www.nationalshareoffice.com

Death and Dying
   http://dying.miningco.com

TAPS: Tragedy Assistance Programs for Survivors of death in the line of military duty
   www.taps.org

# EXAM QUESTIONS

## CHAPTER 8
### Questions 77-86

77. A recommendation to health professionals who help those experiencing chronic sorrow is to be

    a. supportive while comparing the griever to others who have experienced the same type of loss.

    b. empathetic by listening and being supportive while focusing on feelings and the unique needs of the griever.

    c. helpful by not asking questions that could be upsetting.

    d. concerned about services in which volunteers are selected, trained, and supported by professionals.

78. A key question when assessing and planning care of the bereaved is

    a. "can you tell me about what makes the experience easy for you?"

    b. "can you tell me about how you see your future?"

    c. "can you tell me about something other than death?"

    d. "can you tell me about the death, how he/she died?"

79. Groups that are usually based in the community and run by the bereaved, providing an important source of normalization, are called

    a. bereavement counseling.

    b. bereavement self-help groups.

    c. psychoeducational workshops.

    d. normal groups.

80. Those who attend an informational type of bereavement support group are seeking ways to

    a. live their life in a more constructive way.

    b. find help through the Internet.

    c. socialize and meet for bus trips.

    d. create a personal web site

81. Participants in bereavement support groups can become frustrated by the unending talker who dominates the conversation so often that others in the group are

    a. able to listen and offer support.

    b. able to use clichés to help each other cope.

    c. not given the opportunity to share their story.

    d. uneasy, becoming tearful and emotional.

82. A problem with bereavement support groups is the member who takes on the role of captain and attempts to

    a. rescue the group members from their pain of loss.

    b. ignore the group facilitator and to run things.

    c. stop the tears of other members.

    d. dominate the conversation.

83. Online bereavement support groups and networks are open to

    a. adults living in the United States.

    b. adults living in the United States and Canada.

    c. worldwide membership.

    d. individuals who have already posted on boards.

84. The bereaved can find easily accessible social and professional support with positive role models, shared experiences, practical information helper therapy, empowerment, and advocacy efforts in

    a. bereavement support groups.

    b. individual counseling.

    c. houses of worship.

    d. online groups and networks.

85. The overriding goal of a psycho-educational workshop is to

    a. provide support to those who are dying and to those who are present during their last moments.

    b. empower the participants by offering information that guides them in understanding the topic and how it relates to their experience.

    c. share one's story, reach out to others who share similar experiences, and learn their approach to healing.

    d. create a belief in some meaning or order in the world with a higher power as the essence of that belief.

86. Some of the workshops related to drunken driving accidents, heart attacks, natural causes, and suicides take place to

    a. educate survivors as they share their grief with others who have experienced similar types of loss.

    b. take advice of the group over that of their physician.

    c. share their loss with grieving individuals on the Internet.

    d. offer information on time frame, group participation expectations, privacy issues, confidentiality, and group goals.

# CHAPTER 9

# PROFESSIONAL CAREGIVER ISSUES

## CHAPTER OBJECTIVE

After completing this chapter, the reader will understand ways to prevent burnout and compassion fatigue and how to handle particularly difficult end-of-life situations.

## LEARNING OBJECTIVES

After studying this chapter, the reader will be able to

1. differentiate between stress, stressor, and burnout.

2. identify strategies that prevent compassion fatigue.

3. indicate the importance of expressing emotion when dealing with a dying child.

The preceding chapters familiarized the reader with some of the most needed information on providing support to the dying and to those who are grieving. The purpose of this chapter is to expand the reader's knowledge about their own personal issues, burnout, and compassion fatigue.

## ACKNOWLEDGING LOSS

*The formation of a professional self can be and often is quite frightening.*
— M.J. Adolson, 1995, p. 35.

Nurses are committed to providing care and, in so doing, create relationships and bonds with patients and their families. When a patient dies, the nurse experiences a loss. Papadatou (2000) maintains those losses can be grouped into six major categories.

1. Loss of a close relationship with a particular patient with whom one has shared part of a significant journey.

2. Loss due to professional's identification with the pain of family members.

3. Loss of one's unmet goals and expectations and one's professional self-image and role.

4. Losses related to one's personal system of beliefs and assumptions about life.

5. Past unresolved losses or anticipated losses.

6. The death of self
(p.62).

In a sense, after the death of a patient, a nurse has to deal with several losses, and the death of self, can be the most difficult to accept. The nurse may reflect upon the bond shared with a particular patient, but when that patient dies, the nurse is reminded that one day, he or she will die, as well. Therefore, a nurse is reminded of his or her own mortality each time a patient dies. As the nurse attempts to transcend the loss of their patient and find meaning in it, he or she can experience the grief or avoid or repress it. Whether avoiding, expressing, or experiencing grief, a health professional's grieving process is both an individual and social interactive process (see Figure 9-1). The nurse's "sense of self-identity" is tied up in a professional and personal role. When a nurse goes to work, his or her personal self and lifestyle come

## FIGURE 9-1: HEALTH PROFESSIONALS' GRIEVING PROCESS

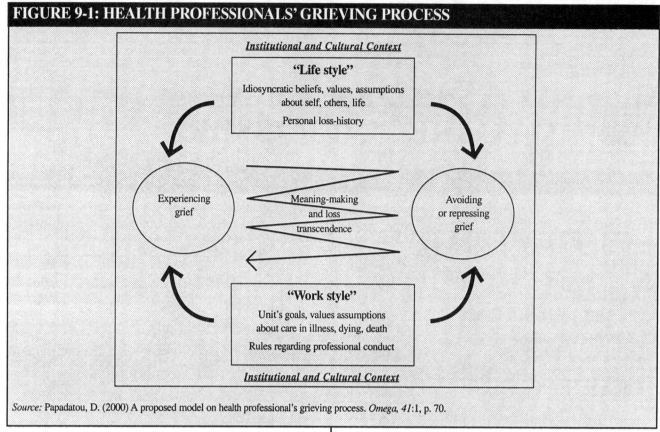

*Source:* Papadatou, D. (2000) A proposed model on health professional's grieving process. *Omega, 41*:1, p. 70.

along. A nurse needs to acknowledge the pain associated with a patient's dying, express their feelings, balance professionalism, respond and work through the loss, and achieve desired goals. If these needs are not met, burnout will be experienced. (Kaplan, 2000, p. 200).

## Stress and Burnout

Stress refers to a physiological reaction or response, regardless of the source, and stressor refers to the stimulus that brings about the stress reaction (Everly & Lating, 2002). Burnout is a state of physical, emotional, and mental exhaustion. The symptoms are caused by the cumulative stress that health professionals experience throughout their careers, which is cumulative and predictable.

> We caregivers believe we are the strong ones. Other people come to us for help. We don't think of ourselves as also vulnerable. Because so much of our sense of self-identity is tied up in our professional roles, to acknowledge an inner sense of dissonance,

a lessening of attachment to the professional role, would mean acknowledging to others that we also have needs (Jevne & Reily-Williams, 1998, p.92).

Does the nurse need to believe that he or she is the strong one? To be strong is to be efficient, not be easily upset, and have physical, moral, and intellectual power. However, the nurse is human, and in being human, is vulnerable. Corr, Nabe, and Corr (2003) note:

> Good helpers need to be open to suggestions and support from other persons—even from the dying person or the family they are helping. Indeed, when dying persons are freed from the burden of distressing symptoms and made to feel secure, they can often be very thoughtful and sensitive in caring for those around them. In short, none of us is without needs in coping with someone else's mortality or with our own mortality. We all can benefit from help as we look to our own tasks in coping (p. 175).

Many nurses have felt tremendous idealism and altruism when first becoming health professionals. We may have become nurses to be instruments of change, to gain respect, to earn a good living, to satisfy a need to heal, or to make a difference in people's lives. This feeling of making a difference in life brings satisfaction.

A nurse is devoted to healing and helping others. Every day the nurse encounters patients and families living through health crisis situations. Peer supervision may help nurses cope with crisis situations. Perhaps the individual had hopes and fantasies about what it would be like to be a nurse. As time passes, the fantasies never come to pass, and the hopes may be dashed. During peer supervision, nurses can address what happened and how they felt before, during, and after the situation.

To maintain a high level of job performance a nurse must be able to effectively cope with the physical, mental, and emotional stress of work and personal life. As shown in the following example, a nurse must be aware of personal issues when providing care.

## Example

Nathan is dying of AIDS. Louise is Nathan's nurse. During Nathan's assessment, Louise realized that she was focusing on her brother's illness and shared her personal problems with Nathan. Though self-disclosure is acceptable, she realized that she was more focused on her brother than the patient. She speaks with her supervisor and together they worked through the problems Louise was facing.

Louise, Nathan's nurse, could meet with a group of nurses every other week or possibly once a month to talk about this case. She can also discuss the triggers, the stimulus that initiates how she responds to the patient. It is the trigger that causes a strong emotional reaction in her that is not about the patient. It is about her brother. With peer supervision, she could discuss her reactions, take herself off the case, or get help while working on the personal life stress of caring for a patient who has the same condition as her brother.

## Sources of Stress

Personal life stress can include major life transitions and medical, family, or money problems. Patient-induced stress includes angry outbursts, accusations of incompetence, suicidal threats, and dysfunctional family members. Work environment stress includes time pressures, excessive caseloads, non-supportive peers, excessive paperwork, lack of resources, and incompetent supervisors.

## Example

Nicholas has been an LPN for 8 years and was once enthusiastic about his work. Through the years he has over-identified with his patients and expended much of his own energy into their care. Lately he feels stagnated and no longer has the desire to be a nurse. He complains of not having enough power in his work and being overworked. He has begun to resent his patients and is thinking about leaving the field he once loved. He now feels bored and detached from his work. Nicholas tells one of the nurses, "I really don't care anymore."

A nurse must also cope with self-induced stress, which may include feelings of perfectionism, fear of failure, and need for approval, as shown in the following example.

## Example

Mary, a nursing home administrator, had always taken great pride in her work. Her residents received quality care, and her staff voiced few complaints. One resident, Mr. Zwirn, had had several issues with the facility and with his care. His family had always wanted meetings with Mary and complained endlessly. They had wanted certain things that simply were not possible. Since Mr. Zwirn's death, Mary has spent more time thinking about this particular resident than all the residents that have been and still are pleased with their care. She feels as though the situation was a failure, and it bothers her a great deal. Mary speaks with a co-worker, who advises her to reflect on what happened, what she could have changed, and what she could learn from the experience that could help her grow. Mary realizes that she was trying to be flexible with the patient and his family but that their demands were not acceptable.

The stress a nurse experiences will worsen if it is not recognized from the very beginning. Past unresolved issues will increase the burden of care. Personal life stress, patient-induced stress, and work environment stress are all likely to occur as nurses provide care to those who are suffering. Kanel (2003) notes:

> Reduced feelings of personal accomplishment have been associated with burnout, so it would appear that one way to reduce burnout would be to spend more time with clients. However, because paperwork is often required in human services occupations, management would be wise to ensure that workers have enough client contact, as this seems to buffer workers against the worst effects of stress and is a valuable source of reward among staff. Other factors that may reduce burnout include workers feeling that they have some control over their time at work, have some control over their workload, and can organize their own work. Recognition of quality of care is also helpful in reducing burnout as is clarity over one's role at work (p. 70).

Both competent nurses and incompetent nurses can experience burnout. Usually, it is a result of being frustrated and not being able to achieve one's goals. Furman (2002) notes that health professionals are at a risk for burnout if they have experienced any of the following during the previous 3 to 6 months.

- Dreaded going to work or stayed late when it wasn't necessary.
- Taken long breaks and lunches or no breaks or lunches.
- Experienced chronic backaches, headaches, or other nagging physical symptoms.
- Felt numb and uninterested in everything.
- Slept restlessly.
- Slept more or less than usual.
- Felt dissatisfied with your life.
- Used alcohol, drugs, food, or sex to escape your feelings.
- Felt irritable, angry, or hostile with your patients or colleagues.
- Spent more time alone or felt withdrawn.
- Felt depressed or emotionally drained.
- Felt as though you're not accomplishing anything with your patients.
- Lost interest in or resented your patients.
- Felt preoccupied with thoughts , images, or circumstances of death, even during your leisure time

(p. 57).

## Burnout Prevention

*After working in community mental health for five years, I was burned out, or burned up, by a sense of hopelessness after overextending myself to help people and no one seemingly appreciated my efforts.*

— M.E. Young, 1997, p. 45

One way to prevent burnout is to maintain one's boundaries. A nurse must set personal and professional boundaries when helping patients in their home. Durkin (2000) recommends four steps to keeping boundaries clear.

1. Stay focused on assisting the patient and family to reach the planned goals and outcomes.

2. Reassure the patient and family that they do not have to become a friend or confidant in order to receive services.

3. Do not share personal problems. It is inappropriate and unfair for visiting staff to share their own issues and concerns.

4. Share any concerns you have with your supervisor. Be comfortable in recounting situations and encounters to validate your impression and to develop approaches

(p. 479).

Professional support groups are also excellent places to discuss boundaries. It is during these group meetings that nurses can address present feelings and personal motives. For example, to make a personal application, ask yourself, "What do I get out of being a nurse?" "Do I feel reasonably competent in my role?" This quick assessment of how you are coping with your role as a nurse can help prevent burnout by making you aware of how you are feeling. Are you losing sight of your professional boundaries?

# COMPASSION FATIGUE

*The capacity for compassion and empathy seems to be at the core of our ability to be wounded by the work.*

— B.H. Stamm, 1995, p.ix

The demands of caring for those dying may eventually take its toll upon anyone's personal and professional life. The term 'compassion fatigue' refers to a state of tension and preoccupation with the individual or cumulative trauma of clients. It has also been called secondary victimization (Figley, 1982). The variety of symptoms include re-experiencing the patient's traumatic event, dread of working with certain people, difficulty separating work from personal life, and guilt for surviving. Figley (2002) maintains:

> In the traumatic situation where victims could not be saved or properly cared for, compassion strain reaches traumatic proportions and may be called compassion fatigue. It includes maladaptive compassion strain, but in addition includes severe anguish and intense guilt associated with the meaning of not having prevented, or even having caused, harm or death. The distress and trauma of not having done enough to avert suffering or death is a common secondary stress and secondary trauma response on helpers (p.26).

Compassion fatigue implies a physical, emotional, and spiritual exhaustion with a decline in ability to experience joy as the body becomes exhausted. Those with compassion fatigue may experience hopelessness, blame, anger, physical fatigue, and drug abuse. They may be irritable and unable to fall asleep. Lack of sleep along with the other symptoms may put not only their job in jeopardy but also their patient's lives. There is a risk for depression, anxiety disorders, or total avoidance by leaving the field of nursing.

A nurse provides compassionate care to those in need. However, as caregivers, nurses can lose sight of their own needs. After working with patients all day or night, the nurse goes home. Before going home, it is a good idea for the nurse to take a few moments to debrief. Debriefing can be done with a few of the other staff members to discuss their day. By debriefing, the vicarious traumatization and cumulative stress will be lessened. Chandler (1999) maintains "hearing the stories, witnessing the grief, may result in a mirror image of those symptoms in care-givers over time" (p. 66). Nurses who discuss their day with others before going home may be at less risk to mirror the symptoms of those in their care.

Nurses who work in disaster situations are also at risk for compassion fatigue. Often, by identifying with those who are suffering, the health professional becomes at risk for compassion fatigue. Parkes (2003) notes,

> You have to get used to working in an atmosphere of fear and anger, to meeting prejudice and hostility from traumatized officials and fellow professionals, and to witness the secondary traumas that so often magnify the effects of the disaster itself (p. 43).

Figley (2002) suggests, "Secondary traumatic stress or compassion stress is a natural by-product of caring for traumatized people, occurring suddenly and without warning, especially in professionals who display great empathic abilities and who tend to identify with their clients' suffering." Though it can occur suddenly and without warning, it can also increase over time.

## Measuring Compassion Satisfaction as Well as Fatigue

An experienced critical care nurse notes, "I say, 'I am only one person' to remind others or myself that it takes many people many days to achieve a difficult goal" (Figley, 2002, p. 217).

Now is the time to personally address stress and possible burnout you are experiencing (see Table 9-1).

Compassion is the caring awareness of another person's anguish and, at the same time, a need to lessen it. If a health professional experiences compassion satisfaction, they may not experience compassion fatigue. There may be a strain between their satisfaction in their role in providing care and the compassion fatigue they feel. In a study by Wee & Myers (2003) measuring compassion satisfaction, compassion fatigue, and critical incident stress management, the authors found that experience, knowledge and maturity play a role in compassion satisfaction. They found that growing older might counter the effects of burnout, perhaps due to the wisdom and experience gained through the years.

Perhaps through their own experience, older nurses realize that they are simply doing the best they can.

## Preventing Compassion Fatigue

If a nurse does not know how she feels after a patient dies, she may be cutting herself off from her feelings.

### Example

Mindy has been an emergency room nurse for six years. During those years she has helped saved countless individuals and has witnessed many deaths. Last month, three children were brought in from a school bus crash. Though the staff worked on the children, all three died in the emergency room. Mindy says, "I really don't know how I feel. I kind of feel like I am shut off from my feelings." Mindy spoke with her supervisor who helped her understand deadening, where she was cutting herself off from her feelings.

> *Personal Insight*
> *If one of your patients died, what feelings or stressors did you experience after the death?*

As a nurse, you may have the difficult task of preparing your patient's body for the morgue. Iserson (1999) notes:

> Once the patient has been pronounced dead, staff start using such words as "the body" or "the corpse," emotionally separating it from the "patients" for whom they must continue caring. In most health care facilities, nurses have another role—preparing bodies for the morgue. A little-discussed element of this job is to clean and remove extraneous medical equipment from the body (if it is not a medical examiner's case, when all disposable medical equipment must stay in place until the forensic examination is completed). Nurses or other staff then may tie the mouth closed, secure the hands so that they do not flop around, and shroud the body (p.219).

## TABLE 9-1: PROFESSIONAL QUALITY OF LIFE (1 OF 2)

### Compassion Satisfaction and Fatigue Subscales - Revision III

Helping others puts you in direct contact with other people's lives. As you probably have experienced, your compassion for those you help has both positive and negative aspects. We would like to ask you questions about your experiences, both positive and negative, as a helper. Consider each of the following questions about you and your current situation. Write in the number that honestly reflects how frequently you experienced these characteristics in the last 30 days.

| 0=Never | 1=Rarely | 2=A Few Times | 3=Somewhat Often | 4=Often | 5=Very Often |
|---|---|---|---|---|---|

_____ 1   I am happy.

_____ 2.  I am preoccupied with more than one person I help.

_____ 3.  I get satisfaction from being able to help people.

_____ 4.  I feel connected to others.

_____ 5.  I jump or am startled by unexpected sounds.

_____ 6.  I feel invigorated after working with those I help.

_____ 7.  I find it difficult to separate my personal life from my life as a helper.

_____ 8.  I am losing sleep over a person I help's traumatic experiences.

_____ 9.  I think that I might have been "infected" by the traumatic stress of those I help.

_____ 10. I feel trapped by my work as a helper.

_____ 11. Because of my helping, I feel "on edge" about various things.

_____ 12. I like my work as a helper.

_____ 13. I feel depressed as a result of my work as a helper.

_____ 14. I feel as though I am experiencing the trauma of someone I have helped.

_____ 15. I have beliefs that sustain me.

_____ 16. I am pleased with how I am able to keep up with helping techniques and protocols.

_____ 17. I am the person I always wanted to be.

_____ 18. My work makes me feel satisfied.

_____ 19. Because of my work as a helper, I feel exhausted.

_____ 20. I have happy thoughts and feelings about those I help and how I could help them.

_____ 21. I feel overwhelmed by the amount of work or the size of my caseload I have to deal with.

_____ 22. I believe I can make a difference through my work.

_____ 23. I avoid certain activities or situations because they remind me of frightening experiences of the people I help.

_____ 24. I plan to be a helper for a long time.

_____ 25. As a result of my helping, I have intrusive, frightening thoughts.

_____ 26. I feel "bogged down" by the system.

_____ 27. I have thoughts that I am a "success" as a helper.

_____ 28. I can't recall important parts of my work with trauma victims.

_____ 29. I am an unduly sensitive person.

_____ 30. I am happy that I chose to do this work.

## TABLE 9-1: PROFESSIONAL QUALITY OF LIFE (2 OF 2)

### RESEARCH INFORMATION — ProQOL - CSF-R-III
### Professional Quality of Life: Compassion Satisfaction and Fatigue Subscales

Please note that research is ongoing on this scale and the following scores should be used as a guide, not confirmatory information. Subscales and cut points are theoretically derived from the data When at all possible, data should be used in a continuous fashion, rather than with cut scores. Cut scores should be used for guidance and comparability of samples, not for diagnostic or confirmatory information.

**Theoretical Score Cut-points (revised 7/12/03)**

Currently, using data (n=400) and theory, the cut scores are set at low (bottom 25%) middle 50% and high (upper 25%). Please note that these scores are subject to further revisions as additional data is gathered. See *ProQOL Score Handout* for an editable, consumer friendly version of the scoring and interpretation. This handout may be used for feedback to research participants.

a. Potential for Compassion Satisfaction: The average score is 37 (SD 7; alpha scale reliability .87). About 25% of people score higher than 41 and about 25% of people score below 32.

b. Risk for Burnout: The average score on the burnout scale is 23 (SD 6.0; alpha scale reliability .72). About 25% of people score above 28 and about 25% of people score below 19.

c. Risk for Compassion Fatigue: The average score on this scale is 13 (SD 6; alpha scale reliability .80). About 25% of people score below 8 and about 25% of people score above 17.

**Self-scorning directions (revised 7/12/03)**

1. Be certain you respond to all items.
2. On some items the scores need to be reversed. Next to your response write the reverse of that score. (i.e. 0=0, 1=5, 2=4, 3=3) Reverse the scores on these 5 items: 1, 4, 15, 17 and 29. 0 is not reversed as its value is always null.
3. Mark the items for scoring:
    a. Put an x by the following 10 items: 3, 6, 12, 16, 18, 20, 22, 24, 27, 30
    b. Put a check by the following 10 items: 1, 4, 8, 10, 15, 17, 19, 21, 26, 29
    c. Circle the following 10 items: 2, 5, 7, 9, 11, 13, 14, 23, 25, 28
4. Add the numbers you wrote next to the items for each set of items and compare on theoretical scores.

**SPSS Scoring (revised 7/12/03)**

Reverse scores on items 1, 4, 15, 17, and 29 before computing sums. Do this by recoding into different variables. Pick the input variable and rename it (i.e. 1r, 4r). Old and new variables will be: 0=0, 1=5, 2=4, 3=3, 4=2, 5=1. While it would seem to necessary to reverse the order of the 0 value, this value is not reversed as the 0 represents the absence of the concept and applies regardless of the order of the remaining numbers.

### Your Scores On The ProQOL: Professional Quality of Life Screening
For more information on the ProQOL, go to http://www.isu.edu/~bhstamm
*Based on your responses, your personal scores are below.*
*If you have any concerns, you should discuss them with a physical or mental health care professional.*

**Compassion Satisfaction** _____

Compassion satisfaction is about the pleasure you derive from being able to do your work well. For example, you may feel like it is a pleasure to help others through your work. You may feel positively about your colleagues or your ability to contribute to the work setting or even the greater good of society. Higher scores on this scale represent a greater satisfaction related your ability to be an effective caregiver in your job.

The average score is 37 (SD 7; alpha scale reliability .87). About 25% of people score higher than 41 and about 25% of people score below 32. If you are in the higher range, you probably derive a good deal of professional satisfaction from your position. If your scores are below 32, you may either find problems with your job, or there may be some other reason-for example, you might derive your satisfaction from activities other than your job.

**Burnout** _____

Most people have an intuitive idea of what burnout is. From the research perspective, burnout is associated with feelings of hopelessness and difficulties in dealing with work or in doing your job effectively. These negative feelings usually have a gradual onset. They can reflect the feeling that your efforts make no difference, or they can be associated with a very high workload or a non-supportive work environment. Higher scores on this scale mean that you are at higher risk for burnout.

The average score on the burnout scale is 23 (SD 6.0; alpha scale reliability .72). About 25% of people score above 28 and about 25% of people score below 19. If your score is below 19, this probably reflects positive feelings about your ability to be effective in your work. If you score above 28, you may wish to think about what at work makes you feel like you are not effective in your position. Your score may reflect your mood; perhaps you were having a "bad day" or are in need of some time off. If the high score persists or if it is reflective of other worries, it may be a cause for concern.

**Compassion Fatigue/Secondary Trauma** _____

Compassion fatigue (CF), also called secondary trauma (STS), and related to Vicarious Trauma (VT) is about your work-related, secondary exposure to extremely stressful events. For example, you may repeatedly hear stories about the traumatic things that happen to other people, commonly called VT. If your work puts you directly in the path of danger, such as being a soldier or humanitarian aide worker, this is not secondary exposure; your exposure is primary. However, if you are exposed to others' traumatic events as a result of your work, such as in an emergency room or working with child protective services, this is secondary exposure. The symptoms of CF/STS are usually rapid in onset and associated with a particular event. They may include being afraid, having difficulty sleeping, having images of the upsetting event pop into your mind, or avoiding things that remind you of the event.

The average score on this scale is 13 (SD 6; alpha scale reliability .80). About 25% of people score below 8 and about 25% of people score above 17. If your score is above 17, you may want to take some time to think about what at work may be frightening to you or if there is some other reason for the elevated score. While higher scores do not mean that you do have a problem, they are an indication that you may want to examine how you feel about your work and your work environment. You may wish to discuss this with your supervisor, a colleague, or a health care professional.

*Source:* http://www.isu.edu/~bhstamm/tests/ProQOL_Score_Handout.doc

Patients, family members, and visitors are usually not aware of the procedures. However, the nurse may experience emotions due to what is seen and done. The nurse may react to the tasks completed while emotionally separating from the patient. Creating a ritual activity may help the nurse emotionally separate from the patient for whom the nurse was caring. Rituals used upon returning home, can include lighting a candle in remembrance of the patient or making a special meal in honor of the patient who died, dedicating money in the patient's memory, or writing a letter to the deceased. These activities can provide the nurse with an opportunity to manage stress.

Whether preparing a body for the morgue or delivering bad news, nurses are at risk for compassion fatigue and will benefit from finding ways to manage their stress. A recent study (Stewart, Lord, & Mercer, 2000) found two strategies death notifiers used to cope with the stress of death notification. These strategies were spending time with their family or talking with their fellow workers. There are some situations that nearly every professional finds emotionally difficult. When such a situation reminds professionals about their own past loss or a loss that might occur to someone they care about, they may experience remembered or anticipatory grief. Though unresolved past loss experiences bring many health professionals into the field, these losses can cause difficulties in the present.

When working with those who are dying and the bereaved, a nurse may experience anticipatory grief over possible future personal losses. In Papadatou's 2000 study, a young nurse reported,

> What consistently happens to me when a child dies is that I think of the death of my father, my brother, the husband I will some day marry or my future children. In every death, I imagine the funeral of my own loved ones (p.63).

As professionals think of these possible future losses and imagine their loved ones dying in the

same way, difficulties may arise. That is why it is important for professionals to find ways to cope with their role in providing support.

As health professionals collectively share information about the patient's care, any interventions done, and their dying, meaning may be found in the death. Awareness of feelings and behaviors after a patient's death is a good step toward interpreting in a symbolic way the meaning of the loss. When that meaning is shared with other health professionals, the interactive process influences each other's reaction and feelings about the loss of the patient. Papadatou (2000) notes that collective and shared meaning is threefold.

- First, it marks and consolidates the passage of a given patient through the unit and sometimes serves as a death ritual.

- Second, it confirms or contradicts the unit's goals, values, and assumptions regarding the care that is provided to dying patients.

- Third, it helps team members to organize and develop their personal stories concerning a patient's death and to share them with other colleagues

(p. 68).

To share the meaning of a patient's death with others is a way to prevent compassion fatigue. While talking about the patient with others, nurses should not lose sight of their intentions while the patient was alive. Nurses who dwell on whether or not they could have done more may feel better simply accepting that what they did was the best that they could do at the time. Talking about their feelings will help. However, there are other strategies that relieve some of the stress after a patient dies. Some of these strategies include interacting with other professionals and colleagues, having a hobby, keeping a journal, talking with a close friend or family member, praying, eating nutritious foods, using guided imagery, exercising, shopping, having breakfast in bed, taking a nap, planning for future enjoyable events, and using humor when appropriate, as shown in the case of Eileen, a nurse in a nursing home.

## Example

Eileen has been a nurse in a nursing home for the past 3 years and has been present for several of the patient's deaths. She makes a point of sharing her feelings with other nurses and finds this practice brings her comfort after a patient's death. Eileen focuses on what she could control and what she could not control. If she finds herself obsessing about certain thoughts, she will talk about them with other nurses. She believes in challenging her own perception of what happened and finds that reviewing her role in the patient's care helps her cope with the patient's death. Eileen keeps a journal. She tries to write in it every few days to help her solve problems, and she finds it reduces her stress. She sometimes dedicates a page to a patient.

## Meditation

Another way to take care of personal needs is to meditate, which refers to focusing, reflecting, or pondering one's thoughts. According to Everly & Lating (2002), while meditating, the individual focuses on one thing, a focal device, and their meditative technique can be categorized by the nature of their focal devices. The authors note four general forms of meditative technique. The first form is mental repetition where the focal device is a word or phrase repeated over and over again (i.e., chanting). The second form is physical repetition where the focal device is focusing awareness on a physical act. (i.e., yoga).

The third form of meditative technique is problem contemplation, where the focal device is attempting to solve a challenging problem and the response to the problem is found in the wisdom and life experience of the person. After the mind is quieted, the individual works on a saying otherwise known as a "koan" but does not actually seek out an answer. Instead, the person resolves the problem through thought (i.e., what is the sound of one hand clapping?)

The fourth form of meditative technique is visual concentration where the focal device is an image (i.e., a relaxing scene or candle flame). A relaxing scene can be found by using guided imagery (GI) to manage the stress at work. Ackerman and Turkoski (2000) notes

> Guided imagery is a technique that can be applied to many situations and can be varied to fit each individual's lifestyle. As nurses, we can help our clients to identify and use coping mechanisms that are both healthy and effective. As individuals, we can help our families, our friends, and ourselves in the same manner. Guided imagery is a technique that, once learned, provides anyone with an intervention with multiple applications (p. 530).

As nurses practice various meditative techniques, they will learn ways to relax. People experience deep relaxation when meditating. Smith (2002) maintains

> The voices of over a thousand research participants suggest the benefits of meditating include:
>
> a. Deeper Perspective (Life has a purpose greater than my personal wants and desires)
>
> b. God (God guides, loves, and comforts me; I put myself in God's hands)
>
> c. Inner Wisdom (I trust the body's wisdom and healing powers; there are sources of strength and healing deep within me)
>
> d. Taking It Easy (Sometimes it is important to know when to stop trying, let go, and relax)
>
> e. Acceptance (Sometimes it is important to accept things that cannot change)
>
> f. Optimism (I believe in being optimistic, both in general and about how well I will deal with current hassles)
> (p. 235).

## Stress Management

Aiken (1994) notes:

To cope with their feelings of frustration, help-lessness, and embarrassment, some doctors and nurses tend to stereotype terminally ill patients as already dead or at least as different from the living. Depersonalization, which is reflected in the tendency to refer to patients by a specific disease and room number rather than a personal name, is most marked when the patient is most helpless (p. 297).

Nurses may have problems with stress management because they are accustomed to a high level of stress. They may think of self-care as selfish and have poor boundaries. Nurses may not have been taught about or developed a role model for stress care. They may develop unhealthy methods for stress release such as over-eating or drinking, over-medication, and uncontrolled anger. To better cope with stress, nurses should begin to monitor themselves for stress daily by using a level of 1 to 10. This gives them a daily reminder of their stress level. By acknowledging that the stress exists, they can then do something about it. To better cope with stress, nurses can develop a stronger sense of self and improve personal boundaries, as they remain safe in their professional roles. They can find a role model of good self-care and develop their own self-care practices. By following these guidelines, nurses will not use unhealthy methods of stress release and will find strength in their role as compassionate caregivers.

The intensity of a nurse's strength comes from a willingness to give to patients. However, nurses must be realistic about what they can achieve. Nurses should acknowledge the painful experiences that occur throughout the day and find ways to process their own grief due to a patient's dying or death. They can continue to provide care to other patients without building up resentment if they know their boundaries and limitations. Rando (1984) notes:

There is also the question of how much of ourselves we are willing or able to give to others. We must acknowledge the fact that sometimes we must only 'be, not do;' we must be realistic about how much we are truly capable of accomplishing for the patient; and we must realize that we can only be usefully involved with a certain number of patients at any one time. If we are not honest about it, we will find ourselves building up resentment towards patients and their families. It is better to acknowledge our limits and be able to provide as much care as we can willingly (p. 441).

Personally, your role as a nurse is an empowering one. Healing those who are ill and supporting those who care for them is not an easy task. As you move forward in your career, ask yourself what you intend to do differently with your patients and their family members and in your personal life so that you do not burn out or experience compassion fatigue.

# PARTICULARLY DIFFICULT SITUATIONS

When children die, they leave behind a part of themselves. The bond between the child and nurse is significant. After the child's death, nurses attempt to find meaning in both the life and death. When nurses care for a dying child, a bond is formed; when that child dies, the nurses respond in their own way. Papadatou (2000) cited these among other responses from nurses and physicians as examples of experiences of treating dying children.

I cry and cry for a week before a death...

And after the death, I sometimes dream of the child and I light a candle, especially if I have not attended the funeral. At home, I withdraw and don't want to talk to anybody, not even to my children. (p. 63).

I'm ashamed because I feel nothing. It's as if I were washing dishes...that's the way I approach the dead patient. I disconnect the child from the machines without feeling a thing. At that very moment, I must be cool... but when the act is over, I may go away and cry. (p.67).

The nurse in the first scenario experienced anticipatory grief, crying for a week before the child dies. It is difficult to cope when actively grieving but not sharing that grief with anyone. Though nurses may create private rituals, sometimes there is no one to communicate with in the family or at work to share feelings about the death. Do nurses, as professionals, feel that it is not appropriate to express grief openly?

The nurse in the second scenario experienced dissociation and feet ashamed in feeling nothing. The nurse mentions, "I must be cool." Why do nurses feel the need to be cool? When does a nurse learn to be cool, and how long does the coolness remain after disconnecting the child from the machines? What are the triggers and what does the word "cool" mean to nurses? The term cool is defined as "steady, dispassionate calmness and self-control, also lacking friendliness and expressing restrained emotion" (Webster's New Collegiate Dictionary, 1977). Nurses may shut off their own feelings during the act of disconnecting the child from the machine. If a nurse "must" be cool and "may" go away and cry, feelings are being shut off. By showing emotion in the presence of the child's parents and family, their shared grief may help them to cope with the difficult task of taking a child off life support.

## The Dying Child's Family

Reilly-Smorawski, Armstrong, and Catlin (2002) studied the relationship between the caregiv-er and the family of a dying baby. The findings provide a basis for asserting that health professionals experience a loss reaction when providing care to those who are dying.

If a grieving parent observed a NICU staff member's tears, that profound recollection was frequently shared with other parents. Being aware of what occurs to each family after the baby's death in the NICU is significant to caregivers; the post-death follow-up may help nurses cope with their feelings of sadness, failure, and spiritual distress accompanying the deaths (Reilly-Smorawski, Armstrong, & Catlin, 2002). The medical team feels a difficult strain, as the dying child symbolizes the most tragic life event (Kaplan, 2000).

Nurses may find it difficult to be objective and professional as the family of the dying child becomes attached to them. Durkin (2000) notes, "Patients and families facing a health crisis or an impending death may intensify the attachment with a care provider who is then challenged to convey a caring, concerned attitude, all the time being objective and professional (p. 478). If a nurse attempts to be objective and professional without expressing emotions in front of the family, stress levels may increase. Some of the grief reactions of the health professionals are similar to those of family members. Papadatou (2000) noted that common grief reactions of health professionals after the repeated deaths of their patients include anger, guilt, and a need to cry as they experience sorrow. Nurses recognize the impact of their participation in the patient's care and may even find relief after the patient's death. However, such nurses' increased stress level can lead to despair, depression, withdrawal from activities and people, and other anxiety disorders, including post-traumatic stress disorder.

## Children's Understanding of Terminal Illness

Bluebond-Langner (1978) has suggested "five stages of understanding that terminally ill children go through, almost regardless of age:"

1. Acquire information that it is a serious illness.

2. Learn the names of drugs and their side effects.

3. Know the purposes of treatments and procedures.

4. Understand the disease as a series of relapses and remissions.

5. On hearing of the death of a peer, they understand the disease as a series of relapses and remissions that will end in death

(p. 166).

The stages described above indicate how children make sense of their terminal illness. What can we learn from the way children understand their situation? We can see that they seek out information, attempt to learn what is happening to them, and that the experience is an ever-changing one. Nurses who care for dying children share similar needs. After a child dies, the nurse will seek out information. If they were not present during the death, nurses will inquire as to how the child died and who was present during the death. They may seek information regarding services and attempt to learn what happened. When a child dies, it is difficult to understand. In learning what happened, the nurse attempts to find meaning in the child's death and, in doing so, experiences grief.

In a study (Papadatou, Papazoglou, Bellali, & Petraki, 2002) of nurses and physicians caring for dying children, findings revealed that both physicians (82%) and nurses (94%) were grieving after the child died. Nurses' reported grief reactions as crying, sadness, anger, recurring thoughts of the dying conditions, and the death. Nurses reported withdrawing into themselves. Unlike physicians, nurses reported sharing their experiences with colleagues for emotional support. Nurses reported

finding meaning in the death, and 75% felt emotionally supported by their colleagues, as the social sharing of grief became a collective experience. Whether a health professional experiences grief or avoids it, their grieving process is influenced by their personal loss history and their work style (Papadatou, 2000).

# SUMMARY

This chapter looked at the scope of professional caregiver issues. Many nurses felt tremendous idealism and altruism when first becoming a health professional, and the chapter explored how that can change as time passes. The chapter examined acknowledging loss. The focus was on the role of personal life stress, patient-induced stress, work environment stress, and self-induced stress in respect to burnout. Burnout prevention was highlighted.

The next part of this chapter examined compassion fatigue and prevention. Ways to measure compassion satisfaction were examined. The chapter also highlighted what a nurse experiences after a patient's death.

The chapter ended by addressing a particularly difficult situation, the nurses' experience of treating dying children. Bluebond-Langner's five stages of understanding what terminally ill children go through, almost regardless of age, and how their dying affects the nurses who care for them were examined.

# RESOURCES

## Professional Caregiver Issues on the Internet

American Academy of Family Physicians
http://www.aafp.org/fpm/20000400/39over.html

Arizona Center for Social Trauma
http://www.acstrauma.com/compassion.htm

The Center for Professional Well-Being
    http://www.cpwb.org/

NurseWeek
    http://www.nurseweek.com/news/features/
    01-11/stress.html

Stress Assess: Online assessment
    http://wellness.uwsp.edu/Health_Service/
    Services/stress.htm

Stress Busters: On the job stress
    http://stressrelease.com/strssbus.html

Thoughts, Links, and Readings on Caregiver
    Stress & Burnout for Medical and
    Psychological professionals, Family
    Caregivers, and Clergy
    http://www.synspectrum.com/healself.html

# EXAM QUESTIONS

## CHAPTER 9
### Questions 87-100

87. Physioological reaction, or response, regardless of the source is called

    a. stressor.

    b. burnout.

    c. stress.

    d. compassion fatigue.

88. The stimulus that serves to bring about the stress reaction is

    a. a stressor.

    b. stress.

    c. secondary traumatic stress.

    d. compassion fatigue.

89. A state of physical, emotional, and mental exhaustion is

    a. meditation.

    b. burnout.

    c. compassion fatigue.

    d. compassion satisfaction.

90. Work environment stress includes

    a. major life transitions.

    b. non-supportive peers.

    c. feelings of perfectionism.

    d. a patient's dysfunctional family members.

91. A state of tension and preoccupation with the individual or cumulative trauma of clients is

    a. burnout.

    b. guided imagery.

    c. compassion satisfaction.

    d. compassion fatigue.

92. A natural by-product of caring for traumatized people that may occur suddenly and without warning is

    a. secondary traumatic stress.

    b. meditation.

    c. burnout.

    d. guided imagery.

93. Experience, knowledge, and maturity play a role in

    a. compassion fatigue.

    b. burnout.

    c. secondary traumatic stress.

    d. compassion satisfaction.

94. A strategy professionals may employ to prevent compassion fatigue is

    a. giving up a hobby.

    b. not sharing their feelings with close friends or family members.

    c. interacting with other professionals and colleagues.

    d. not planning for future enjoyable events.

95. Focusing, reflecting, or pondering one's thoughts is part of

   a. burnout.

   b. meditation.

   c. compassion fatigue.

   d. compassion satisfaction.

96. When providing care to those who are dying, professionals may experience a

   a. hope reaction.

   b. coping reaction.

   c. loss reaction.

   d. symbolic reaction.

97. For those parents who had witnessed the tears of an NICU staff member, it

   a. made their grief more difficult to process.

   b. was a profound memory they often shared with others.

   c. caused additional stress.

   d. resulted in their being more upset.

98. The medical team feels a difficult strain, as the dying child symbolizes

   a. objectiveness and professionalism.

   b. their own death.

   c. the difficult task of taking a child off life-support.

   d. the most tragic life event.

99. A nurse may find it difficult to be objective and professional as the family of the dying child

   a. expresses emotions.

   b. finds relief after the patient's death.

   c. becomes attached to them.

   d. withdraws from activities and people.

100. After a child dies, a nurses' grief reaction includes

   a. knowing the purpose of treatment and options.

   b. keeping feelings from colleagues.

   c. crying, sadness, and anger.

   d. denial that the death took place.

**This concludes the final examination.**

# GLOSSARY

**active euthanasia:** Otherwise known as assisted suicide or assisted death. An act is committed where the patient administers a death-causing agent to end his or her life with the assistance of someone who provides the means. Also, the deliberate ending of a life, as in putting an animal "to sleep."

**accepted assisted suicide:** When a patient requests assistance in dying and the physician does not explore alternatives and few, if any, options are discussed.

**acute care setting:** A type of institution (i.e., hospital) that emphasizes assessment and diagnosis of illness and disease together with cure-oriented interventions for reversible or correctable conditions.

**acute phase:** Initiated by the diagnosis of a life-threatening illness, where an individual attempts to understand the disease, maximize health, develop coping strategies, explore effects of diagnosis, express feelings, and integrate present reality into a sense of past and future.

**advance directive:** An oral or written instruction about a person's future medical treatment in case they become unable to speak for themselves.

**altruistic suicide:** Individuals who complete suicide because they are deeply integrated into a social group, believe it is their duty to die for that group, and their death benefits the entire group.

**anomic suicide:** An individual who, in a crisis situation, does not see any solution to the problem, believes their life has no value in their society, and kills themself.

**anticipatory mourning:** Mourning that arises before the actual death in the anticipation of a future loss and is a form of normal grief.

**bereavement:** The time period after a death that emcompasses the adjustment to living without the person who died.

**bereavement self-help group:** A support group that offers mutual aid; support systems for the bereaved run by the bereaved.

**body donation:** Where the body is donated to medical science.

**brain death:** Characterized by the end of all brain activity, complete unresponsiveness, and no spontaneous breathing.

**burnout:** A state of physical, emotional, and mental exhaustion caused by the cumulative stress that health professionals experience through their careers.

**capable:** A determination in the opinion of a court, or in the opinion of the patient's attending physician or consulting physician, psychiatrist, or psychologist, that a patient has the ability to make and communicate health care decisions to health care providers, including communication through persons familiar with the patient's manner of communicating if those persons are available.

**cardiac death:** The moment the heart stops beating.

**causality:** The origins of actions or consequences.

**cell death:** Death of individual body cells.

**chronic phase:** A grief stage that involves managing the symptoms and side effects of bereavement while carrying out health regimes, normalizing life, maximizing social support, expressing feelings, and finding meaning in the suffering.

**clinical social worker:** A health care worker who has at least a master's degree in social work and two years' experience in a clinical setting. They counsel those with emotional problems and also arrange for needed social services.

**closed awareness:** When patient does not know he or she is dying.

**compassion:** The caring awareness of another person's anguish and, at the same time, a need to lessen it.

**compassion fatigue:** A state of tension and preoccupation with the individual or cumulative trauma of clients, also called secondary victimization.

**complicated mourning:** Mourning intensified, extended, or altered by pressing concerns.

**communication:** The ability to understand and be understood.

**cremation:** From the Latin word cremo, which means "to burn." The process of reducing the human body to bone fragments using high heat and flame.

**culture:** A way of life that represents a specific group of people and includes all of their customs, beliefs, values, and attitudes.

**death notification:** The act of informing significant others their loved one is dead.

**delayed grief:** When a significant period of time elapses between the loss and the onset of grief reaction.

**discussed assisted suicide:** The act of taking one's life after a physician discusses alternatives and encourages the individual to look at all of his or her options.

**disenfranchised grief:** Grief that persons experience when they incur a loss that is not or cannot be openly acknowledged, publicly mourned, or socially supported

**donation:** The act of giving one's organs or tissue to someone else.

**Do Not Resuscitate (DNR):** An advance directive that includes a written request not to have cardiopulmonary resuscitation (CPR).

**Durable Power of Attorney for Health Care:** A type of advance directive that allows the individual to name a representative to make health care decisions on their behalf.

**dying trajectory:** Charting the patient's condition as time passes by setting up a graph with time along the horizontal axis and nearness to death along the vertical axis. The curve is the dying trajectory.

**egotistic suicide:** Individuals who complete suicide due to not having social ties, lacking social integration in society, and isolating themselves.

**embalming:** Preserving the body by removing the blood and replacing it with formaldehyde.

**encouraged assisted suicide:** When the physician encourages the suicide and may provide the means to end the individual's life.

**entombment:** When the body is placed in an above-ground mausoleum.

**eulogy:** A written tribute or speech that is given to commemorate a person who has died.

**euphemism:** A word or phrase that appears to be more pleasant than a particular word being avoided.

**euthanasia:** An active form of mercy killing.

**fatalistic suicide:** Individuals who complete suicide because they consider themselves not to have a future due to political or economic oppression.

**final arrangements:** The care and disposition of a human body and the ceremony following death.

**final disposition:** Management of human remains via burial, cremation, entombment, or body donation.

**Five Wishes:** A document that addresses the person's medical treatment, personal, emotional and spiritual needs and encourages discussing the wishes with the family and physician.

**functional death:** Death occurring when there is an end to all vital functions.

**grief:** A process that includes intense physical, emotional, and spiritual suffering after a loss.

**Health Care Proxy:** A document that allows the patient to appoint someone they trust to make decisions about their medical care if they are incapacitated.

**homicide:** When one person kills another person, recognized as a criminal act even if no body or weapon is found.

**hospice:** Formerly a word used to welcome travelers and the sick; now a philosophy that emphasizes palliative inpatient and home care for terminally ill individuals.

**informed consent:** The process of gaining a patient's permission for a procedure, where the physician involves the patient, informs them of their condition and the risks involved in treatment, and offers them choices.

**instrumental griever:** Individuals who express their grief through a behavior or activity are instrumental grievers. They describe their grief in physical or cognitive terms.

**intuitive griever:** Individuals who express their grief affectively are intuitive grievers. They express their feelings and seek support.

**irreversibility:** The understanding that death is final and, once dead, a person cannot become alive again.

**landmarks:** Important moments or achievements where the terminally ill person completes their affairs and relationships, has a sense of meaning in their life, experiences love of self and others, acknowledges the finality of life and a sense of a new self, and lets go.

**linking objects:** Items that once belonged to the decease that the bereaved now owns. In taking ownership, the significance of the items becomes important.

**Living Will:** An advance directive in which an individual indicates their wishes about the kinds of medical treatments they would accept or reject in different situations if unable to speak for themselves.

**local death:** Death of a part of the body.

**meditate:** Refers to focusing, reflecting, or pondering one's thoughts, where individuals focus on one thing.

**mental health counselor:** Psychologist, psychiatric nurse, certified social worker, certified counselor, licensed therapist, or a person who has a Master's degree in Psychology who provides therapeutic intervention.

**mourning:** The social expressions of grief; grief practices shared by a given cultural group.

**mutual pretense:** When the patient, family, and staff pretend they do not know the patient's prognosis.

**near-death experience:** When pulse and breathing have stopped but the person is resuscitated and survives.

**non-functionality:** The understanding that all life-sustaining functions cease with death.

**open awareness:** When a patient is aware of his or her death and prepares for it and discusses it.

**palliative care:** Enhancing the patient's well-being in the last stages of life, including pain management and a variety of social supports.

**passive euthanasia:** An avoidable death that involves omission of an act. Medical staff in this case sometimes withhold oxygen or end intravenous feedings to those who are terminally ill.

**Patient Self-Determination Act:** Federal law that requires a health agency, hospital, skilled nursing facility, or hospice program to inform all adult patients about their rights to accept or refuse treatment and the right to execute an advance directive.

**permanent memorials:** Lasting impressions and acknowledgements at the site of a death or designated place.

**personal mortality:** Related to universality but reflective of the deeper understanding that not only do all living things die, but that "I will die."

**physician-assisted suicide:** Ending a patient's life when the physician provides the means, such as giving the patient information on how to end their life, prescribing medication or giving the patient equipment.

**postvention:** Those things done that serve to mollify the after-effects for a person who has attempted suicide; also dealing with the adverse effects on the survivor-victims after a person has committed suicide.

**prediagnostic phase:** The time when the individual suspects that he or she is sick and seeks out medication.

**psychiatric nurse-specialist:** Nurses who are certified to work in psychiatric settings.

**psychiatrists:** Medical doctors trained to specialize in mental disorders and prescribe drugs.

**psychologist:** Not physicians, but PhDs who treat individuals by using psychological technique. Since they do not prescribe drugs, they usually do not treat disorders that are caused by abnormal brain chemistry.

**psycho-educational workshops:** Workshops that offer information, opportunities for understanding, and support to the bereaved to impart new knowledge and skills in death, dying, and bereavement situations.

**rational suicide:** Taking one's own life: when the individual possesses a realistic assessment of their situation, the mental processes leading to the decision to commit suicide are unimpaired by psychological illness or severe emotional distress, and the motivational basis for the decision would be understandable to a majority of uninvolved observers from their community or social group.

**recovery phase:** When disease has been cured or the individual is in remission.

**rituals:** Ceremonial actions that have meaning and significance to the individual performing the act.

**social support:** Social caring offered after a death; when the bereft believes there is at least one person who will take the time to listen nonjudgmentally to them while they openly and honestly express their thoughts, feelings, and grief.

**spiritual death:** When the soul, as defined by various religions, departs the body.

**stress:** Refers to a physiological response.

**stressor:** Refers to the stimulus that serves to bring about the stress response.

**suicide threat:** An expressed intention to take one's own life; may be spoken or unspoken, does not involve a self-harmful act but the intention is to communicate that a specific act of self-harm may happen soon.

**suspected awareness:** When a dying patient suspects that others know and attempts to find out more information about his or her prognosis.

**symbolic representation:** A process wherein possessions, creations, or shared experienced of the deceased are imbued with the spirit or memories of the dead.

**terminal disease:** A medically confirmed incurable and irreversible disease that will, within reasonable medical judgment, cause death within 6 months.

**terminal phase:** When an individual copes with impending death by managing pain, symptoms, health procedures and institutional stress.

**thanatology:** A term derived from the name of the Greek god of death, it is a discipline concerned with death and dying.

**traumatic loss:** Deaths that occur beyond the normal range of experience such as a child's death or death that is sudden, unanticipated, and preventable.

**universality:** The understanding that death is inevitable to living things and that all living things die.

**voluntary active euthanasia:** When a clearly competent patient makes a voluntary request of a physician to administer a lethal dose of medication to end the patient's life.

**Werther effect:** The significance of imitative suicidal behavior.

# BIBLIOGRAPHY

Ackerman, C.J. & Turkoski, B. (2000). Using guided imagery to reduce pain and anxiety. *Home Healthcare Nurse, 18*(8), 524-530.

Adachi, K., Bertman, S., Corr, C., Cory, J., Doka, K., Gilbert, K., et al. — International Work Group on Death, Dying, and Bereavement. (2002). Assumptions and principles about psychosocial aspects of disasters. *Death Studies, 26*, 449-462.

Adolson, M.J. (1995). Clinical supervision of therapists with difficult-to-treat patients. *Bulletin of the Menninger Clinic, 59*, 32-52.

Aguilera, D.C. (1998). *Crisis intervention: theory and methodology.* New York: Mosby.

Aiken, L.R. (1994). *Dying, death, and bereavement* (3rd ed.). Boston: Allyn and Bacon.

Alaeddini, J., Julliard, K., Shah, A., Islam, J., & Mayor, M. (2000). Physician attitudes toward palliative care at a community teaching hospital. *The Hospice Journal, 15*(2), 67-86.

Amella, E.J. (2003). Geriatrics and palliative care: Collaboration for quality of life until death. *Journal of Hospice and Palliative Nursing, 5*(1), 40-48.

American Association of Suicidology. (2003). *U.S.A. suicide: 2001 official final data.* Retrieved October 8, 2003 from http://www.suicidology.org/associations/1045/files/2001datapg.pdf

American Association of Suicidology. (2003). *The links between depression and suicide.* Washington, D.C. Retrieved March 15, 2004 from http://www.suicidology.org/displaycommon.cfm?an=1&subarticlenbr=31

Anderson, R.N. (2002). Deaths: Leading causes for 2000. *National Vital Statistics Reports, 50*(16), September 16, 2002. Retrieved August 8, 2003, from http://www.cdc.gov/nchs/data/nvsr/nvsr50/nvsr50_16.pdf

Arias, E. & Smith, B.L. (2003). Deaths: Preliminary data for 2001. *National Vital Statistics Reports, 51*(5), March 14, 2003.

Asinof, E. (1971). *Craig and Joan: Two lives for peace.* New York: Viking.

Attig, T. (1996). *How we grieve: Relearning the world.* NY: Oxford University Press.

Babler, J.E. (1997). A comparison of spiritual care provided by hospice social workers, nurses, and spiritual care professionals. *The Hospice Journal, 12*(4), 15-27.

Balk, D.E. & Corr, C.A. (1996). Adolescents, developmental tasks, and encounters with death and bereavement. In C.A. Corr & D.E. Balk (Eds.), *Handbook of adolescent death and bereavement* (p. 3-24). New York: Springer.

Barrett, T.W. & Scott, T.B. (1989). Development of the grief experience questionnaire. *Suicide and Life-Threatening Behavior, 19*(2), 201-213.

Bantam Books. (2000). *The Bantam Medical Dictionary,* (3rd rev. ed.). New York: Bantam.

Benight, C.C., Flores, J., & Tashiro, T. (2001). Bereavement coping self-efficacy in cancer widows. *Death Studies, 25*, 97-125.

Benoliel, J.Q. (2001). Thanatology and human rights. *Illness, Crisis & Loss, 9*, 8-14.

Bern-Klug, M., DeViney, S., & Ekerdt, D.J. (2000). Variations in funeral-related costs of older adults and the type of pre-need funeral contracts and type of disposition. *Omega, 41*, 23-38.

Biblarz, A., Biblarz, D., Baldree, B., & Pilgrim, M. (1991). Media influence on attitudes toward suicide. *Suicide & Life-Threatening Behavior, 21*, 374-384.

Bluebond-Langner, M. (1978). *The private worlds of dying children.* Princeton, NJ: Princeton University Press.

Boerner, K. & Heckhausen, J. (2003). To have and have not: Adaptive bereavement by transforming mental ties to the deceased. *Death Studies 27*, 199-226.

Bookwala, J., Coppola, K.M., Fagerlin, A., Ditto, P.H., Danks, J.H., & Smucker, W. D. (2001). Gender differences in preferences for life-sustaining treatments and end-of-life values. *Death Studies, 25*, 127-149.

Bowlby, J. (1982). *Attachment* (2nd ed.). New York: BasicBooks.

Brinson, S.V. & Brunk, Q. (2000). Hospice family caregivers: An experience in coping. *The Hospice Journal, 15*(3) 2000, 1-12.

Brock, D.B., Holmes, M.B., Foley, D.J., & Homes, D. (1992). Methodological issues in a survey of the last days of life. In R.B. Wallace & R.F. Woolson (Eds.), *The epidemiological study of the elderly* (p. 315-332). New York: Oxford University Press.

Brock, D.W. (1992). Voluntary active euthanasia. *Hastings Center Report,* March/April 1992, pp. 11-12, 14-17, 19-21.

Bull, M. A., Clark, S., & Duszynski, K. (2002-2003). Lessons from a community's response to the death of Diana, Princess of Wales. *Omega, 46*, 35-49.

Burkholder, G.J., Harlow, L.L., & Washkwich, J.L. (1999). *Journal of Applied Biobehavioral Research, 4*, 1, 27-44.

Bush, G.W. (2003). National Donate Life Month — A Proclamation. Washington, D.C.: Office of the Press Secretary. Retrieved October 17, 2003 from http://www.whitehouse.gov/news/releases/2003/04/20030402.html.

Byock, I. (1996). The nature of suffering and the nature of opportunity at the end of life. *Clinics in Geriatric Medicine, 12*(2), 237-251.

Centers for Disease Control and Prevention; National Center for Injury Prevention and Control. *Suicide in the United States.* Retrieved October 7, 2003 from http://www.cdc.gov/ncipc/factsheets/suifacts.htm.

Chandler, E. (1999). Spirituality. *The Hospice Journal, 14*(3/4), 63-74.

Childs, M. (2000). My privilege. *Nursing 2000, 30*(9), 49-50.

Chin, A.E., Hedberg, K., Higginson, G.K. & Fleming, D.W. (1999). Oregon's Death with Dignity Act: The first year's experience. DHS Salem, OR: Oregon Department of Human Services. Retrieved August 8, 2003, from http://www.dhs.state.or.us/publichealth/chs/pas/year1/pas-rpt.pdf

Cicirelli, V.G. (2001). Personal meanings of death in older adults and young adults in relation to their fears of death. *Death Studies, 25*, 663-683.

Coleman, C.L. (1993). The influence of mass media and interpersonal communication on societal and personal risk judgments. *Communication Research, 20*, 611-628.

Committee on Care at the End of Life. (1997). Chapter 3. In M.J. Field & C.K. Cassel (Eds.), *Approaching death: Improving care at the end of life* (p. 50-86). Washington, DC: National Academy of Sciences. Available online: http://www.nap.edu/readingroom/books/approaching/box3.4.html

Connor, S.R. (1999). New initiatives transforming hospice care. *The Hospice Journal, 14*(3/4), 193-203.

Conwell, Y. (2001). Suicide in later life: A review and recommendations for prevention. *Suicide and Life-Threatening Behavior, 31*(supplement), 32-47.

Corr, C.A., (1995). Children's understanding of death: Striving to understand death. In K.J. Doka (Ed.), *Children mourning, mourning children* (p. 3 -16). Washington, D.C.: Hospice Foundation of America.

Corr, C. A. & Balk, D. E. (Eds.). (1996). *Handbook of adolescent death and bereavement*. New York: Springer.

Corr, C.A., Nabe, C.M., & Corr, D. M. (2000). *Death and dying, Life and living* (3rd ed). Belmont, CA: Wadsworth.

Corr, C.A., Nabe, C.M., & Corr, D. M. (2003). *Death and dying, Life and living* (4th ed.). Belmont, CA: Wadsworth.

Couldrick, A. (1995). A cradling of a different sort. In S.C. Smith & M. Pennells (Eds.), *Interventions with bereaved children* (p. 107-120). London: Jessica Kingsley.

Danforth, M.M. & Glass, Jr., J.C. (2001). Listen to my words, give meaning to my sorrow: A study in cognitive constructs in middle-age bereaved widows. *Death Studies, 25*, 513-529.

Dannemiller. H.C. (2002). The parents' response to a child's murder. *Omega, 45*, 1-21.

Darwin, F. (Ed.). (1887). *The life and letters of Charles Darwin, vol. 1*. (2001). New York City, Appleton.

D'Augelli, A.R., Hershberger, S.L., & Pilkington, N.W. (2001). Suicidality patterns and sexual orientation-related factors among lesbian, gay, and bisexual youths. *Suicide and Life-Threatening Behavior, 31*, 250-264.

DeMong, S.A. (1997). Provision of recreational activities in hospices in the United States. *The Hospice Journal, 12*(4), 57-67.

Denning, D.G., Conwell, Y., King, D., & Cox, C. (2000). Method choice, intent, and gender in completed suicide. *Suicide and Life-Threatening Behavior, 30*, 282-288.

DePaola, S.J., Griffin, M., Young, J., & Neimeyer, R.A. (2003). Death anxiety and attitudes toward the elderly and older adults: The role of gender and ethnicity. *Death Studies, 27*, 335-354.

Department of Health & Human Services — First Gov. Organ donation frequently asked questions. Retrieved October 11, 2003 from http://www.organdonor.gov/faq.html#10

Department of Health & Human Services, National Institute of Mental Health. (2000). Fact Sheet: Schizophrenia research. NIMH Publication No. 00-4500, May 2000.

DeSpelder, L.A. & Strickland, A.L. (2002). *The last dance: Encountering death and dying* (6th ed.). Boston: McGraw Hill.

de Vries, B., Blieszner, R., & Blando, J.A. (2002). The many forms of intimacy, the many faces of grief and intimacy in later life. In K.J. Doka (Ed.), *In living with grief: Loss in later life* (p. 225-242). Washington, D.C.: Hospice Foundation of America.

Dickinson, G.E., Leming, M.R., & Mermann, A.C. (Eds.). (1994). *Dying, death, and bereavement* (2nd ed). Guilford, CT: Dushkin.

Dickinson, G.E., Lancaster, C.J., Clark, D., Ahmedzai, S.H., & Noble, W. (2002). U.K. physicians' attitudes toward active voluntary euthanasia and physician-assisted suicide. *Death Studies, 26*, 479-490.

Doka, K.J. (1989). *Disenfranchised grief: Recognizing hidden sorrow.* Lexington, MA: Lexington Books.

Doka, K.J. (1995-1996). Coping with life threatening illness: A task model. *Omega, 32*(2), 111-122.

Doka, K.J. (2002). *Living with grief: Loss in later life.* Washington, D.C.: Hospice Foundation of America.

Doka, K.J. (2003). What makes a tragedy public? In M. Lattanzi-Licht & K.J. Doka (Eds.). *Living with grief. Coping with public tragedy* (p. 179-189). Washington, D.C.: Hospice Foundation of America.

Donatelle, R.J. (2003). *Health: The basics* (5th Ed.). San Francisco: Benjamin Cummings.

Donnelly, E.F., Field, N.P., & Horowitz, M.J. (2000-2001). Expectancy of spousal death and adjustment to conjugal bereavement. *Omega, 42*, 195-208.

Dorwart, R. A. & Ostacher, M.J. (1999). A community psychiatry approach to preventing suicide. In D.G. Jacobs (Ed.), *The Harvard Medical School guide to suicide assessment and intervention* (p. 52-71). San Francisco: Jossey-Bass.

Dowd, S.B., Poole, V.L., Davidhizar, R., & Giger, J.N. (1998). Death, dying, and grief in a transcultural context: Application of the Giger and Davidhizar assessment model. *The Hospice Journal, 13*, (4), 33-56.

Durkheim, É. (1897). Il suicidio dal punto di vista sociologico. Rivista italiana di sociologia 1: 17-27.

Durkheim, E. (1897). *Le Suicide.* Paris: Presses Universitaires de France. Reissued in 1981.

Durkheim, Emile. (1951). *Suicide: A study in suicidology.* J.A. Spaulding & G. Simpson, Trans. New York: Free Press of Glenco. (Originally published in 1897).

Durkin, N. (2000). The importance of setting boundaries in home care and hospice nursing. *Home Healthcare Nurse, 18*(7), 478-481.

Dyregrov, K., Nordanger, D., & Dyregrov, A. (2003). Predictors of psychosocial distress after suicide, SIDS, & accidents. *Death Studies, 27*, 143-165.

Eakes, G.C., Burke, M.L., & Hainsworth, M.A. (1999). Chronic sorrow: The experiences of bereaved individuals, *Illness, Crisis & Loss, 7*, 172-182.

Elasmar, M., Hasegawa, K., & Brain, M. (1999). The portrayal of women in US prime-time television. *Journal of Broadcasting and Electronic Media, 43*, 20-21.

Ellis, V., Hill, J., & Campbell, H. (1995). Hospice techniques: Strengthening the family unit through the healing power of massage. *The American Journal of Hospice & Palliative Care, 12*(5), 19-21.

Ellis, J.B. & Stump, J.E. (2000). Parents' perceptions of their children's death concept. *Death Studies, 24*, 65-71.

Emanuel, E.J. (1999). What is the great benefit of legalizing euthanasia or physician-assisted suicide? *An International Journal of Social, Political and Legal Philosophy, 109*, 629-642.

Engler, A.J. & Lasker, J.N. (2000). Predictors of maternal grief in the year after a newborn death. *Illness, Crisis & Loss, 8*, 227-243.

Etzersdorfer, E. & Sonneck, G. (1998). Preventing suicide by influencing mass-media reporting: The Viennese experience 1980-1996. *Archives of Suicide Research, 30*(3), 283-312.

Everly, G.S. & Lating, J.M. (2002). *A clinical guide to the treatment of the human stress response* (2nd ed). New York: Kluwer Academic/ Plenum.

Fauri, D.P., Ettner, B., & Kovacs, P. (2000). Bereavement services in acute care settings. *Death Studies, 24*, 51-64.

Feifel, H. & Strack, S. (2001). Thanatologists view death: A 15-year perspective. *Omega, 43*, 97-111.

Fenton, W.S. (2000). Depression, suicide, and suicide prevention in schizophrenia. *Suicide and Life-Threatening Behavior, 30*, 34-49.

Ferrell, B., Coyne, P., & Uman, G. (2000). End-of-life care: Nurses speak out. *Nursing2000, 30*(7), 54-57.

Ferszt, G.C., Massotti, E., Williams, J., & Miller, J.R. (2000). The impact of an art program on an inpatient oncology unit. *Illness, Crisis & Loss, 8*, 189-199.

Figley, C.R. (1982). *Traumatization and comfort: Close relationships may be hazardous to your health.* Keynote presentation at the Conference on Families and Close Relationships: Individuals in Social Interaction. Texas Tech University, Lubbock, TX.

Figley, C.R. (Ed.) (1995). *Compassion fatigue: Coping with secondary traumatic stress disorder in those who treat the traumatized.* New York: Brunner/Mazel.

Figley, R. (2002). Epilogue. In C.R. Figley, *Treating compassion fatigue* (pp. 213-218). Philadelphia: Brunner/Mazel.

Fiske, A. & Arbore, P. (2000). Future directions in late life suicide prevention. *Omega, 42*, 37-53.

Fleming, S. & Balmer, L. (1996). Bereavement in adolescence. In C. A. Corr & D. E. Balk (Eds.), *Handbook of adolescent death and bereavement,* (chapter 7). New York: Springer.

Foley, D.J., Miles, T.P., Brock, D.B., & Philips, C. (1995). Recounts of elderly deaths: Endorsements for the Patient Self-Determination Act. *Gerontologist, 35*(1): 119-121.

Foley, K.M. (2000). Senate Committee on the Judiciary, Hearing entitled, "H.R. 2260, Pain Relief Promotion Act." Retrieved on March 11, 2004, from http://judiciary.senate.gov/old-site/42520kf.htm

Foliart, D.E., Clausen, M., & Siljestrom, C. (2001). Bereavement practices among California hospices. *Death Studies, 25*, 461-467.

Fox, S.S. (1988). *Good grief: Helping groups of children when a friend dies.* Boston: The New England Association.

Friedrichs, J., Daly, M.I., & Kavanaugh, K. (2000). Follow-up of parents who experience a perinatal loss: Facilitating grief and assessing for grief complicated by depression. *Illness, Crisis & Loss, 8*, 296-309.

Fulton, R. & Fulton, J.A. (1971). A psychosocial aspect of terminal care: Anticipatory grief. *Omega, 2*, 91-99.

Furman, J. (2001). Living with dying: How to help the family caregiver. *Nursing2001, 31*(4), 37-41.

Furman, J. (2002). What you should know about chronic grief: Learning to deal with your own lingering emotions when a patient dies. *Nursing 2002, 32*(2), 56-57.

Gadberry, J.H. (2000). When is a funeral not a funeral? *Illness, Crisis & Loss, 8,* 166-180.

Gajdos, K.C. (2002). The intergenerational effects of grief and trauma. *Illness, Crisis & Loss,* 304-317.

Gamino, L.A. Sewell, K.W., & Easterling, L.W. (2000). Scott and White Grief Study—Phase 2: Toward an adaptive model of grief. *Death Studies, 24,* 633-660.

Gamino, L.A., Hogan, N.S., & Sewell, K.W. (2002). Feeling the absence: A content analysis from the Scott and White Grief Study. *Death Studies, 26*, 793-813.

Gensch, B.K. & Midland, D. (2000). When a baby dies: A standard of care. *Illness, Crisis & Loss, 8*, 286-295.

Geron, Y., Ginzburg, K., & Solomon, Z. (2003). Predictors of bereaved parents' satisfaction with group support: An Israeli perspective. *Death Studies, 27*, 405-426.

Gibb, B.E., Alloy, L.B., Abramson, L.Y., Rose, D.T., Whitehouse, W.G., & Hogan, M.E. (2001). Childhood maltreatment and college students' current suicidal ideation: A test of the hopeless theory. *Suicide and Life-Threatening Behavior, 31*, 405-415.

Gilbar, O. & Eden, A. (2000). Suicide tendency in cancer patients. *Omega, 42*(2), 159-170.

Gilbar, O. & Cohen, B.Z. (1995). Oncologists' attitudes to treatment of cancer patients. *Death Studies, 19*, 303-313.

Gilbert, K.R. (2002). Taking a narrative approach to grief research: Finding meaning in stories, *Death Studies, 26*, 223-239.

Glaser, B. & Strauss, A. (1965). *Awareness of dying.* Chicago: Aldine.

Glaser, B. & Strauss, A. (1968). *Time for dying.* Chicago: Aldine.

Gostin, L.O. (1997). Health law and ethics: Deciding life and death in the courtroom. *The Journal of the American Medical Association, 278*, 1523-1528.

Grout, L.A. & Romanoff, B.D. (2000). The replacement child myth. *Death Studies, 24*, 93-113.

Gutierrez, P.M., Rodriguez, P.J. & Garcia, P. (2001). Suicide risk factors for young adults: Testing a model across ethnicities. *Death Studies, 25*, 319-340.

Haddad, A.M. (1992). Ethical problems in home health care. *Journal of Nursing Administration, 22*(3), 46-51.

Hampl, P. (1995). *Burning bright: An anthology of sacred poetry.* New York: Ballantine Books.

Harrold, J.K. (1998). Pain, symptoms, and suffering: Possibilities and barriers. *The Hospice Journal, 13*(1/2) 37-40.

Hatton, R. (2003). Homicide bereavement counseling: A survey of providers. *Death Studies, 27*, 427-448.

Hedtke, L. (2002). Reconstructing the language of death and grief. *Illness, Crisis & Loss, 10*(4), 285-293.

Helming, B. (2001). Unforgettable patient: Lessons from the heart. *Nursing2001, 31*(9), 44-45.

Hendin, H. (1998). *Seduced by death: Doctors, patients, and assisted suicide.* New York: W.W. Norton.

Herkert, B.M. (2000). Communicating grief. *Omega, 41*, 93-115.

Higgins, M.P. (2002). Parental bereavement and religious factors. *Omega, 45*(2) 187-207.

Hines-Smith, S. (2002). "Fret no more my child... For I'm all over heaven all day:" Religious beliefs in the bereavement of African-American, middle-aged daughters coping with the death of an elderly mother. *Death Studies, 26*, 309-323.

Hinton, J. (2003). Exploring and mapping a borderland. *Illness, Crisis & Loss, 1*, 25-36.

Hirshfield, R. & Russell, J. (1997). Assessment and treatment of suicidal patients. *New England Journal of Medicine, 337*, 910-915.

Hogan, N.S., Greenfield, D.B., & Schmidt, L.A. (2001). Development and validation of the Hogan grief reaction checklist. *Death Studies, 25*, 1-32.

Hogan, N.S. & Schmidt, L.A. (2002). Testing the grief to personal growth model using structural equation modeling. *Death Studies, 26*, 615-634.

Holtkamp, S.C. (2000). Anticipatory mourning and organ donation. In T.A. Rando (Ed.), *Clinical dimensions of anticipatory mourning: Theory and practice in working with the dying, their loved ones, and their caregivers* (pp. 511-535). Champaign, IL: Research Press.

Horowitz, M.J., Siegel, B., Holen, A., Bonnano, G.A., Milbrath, C., & Stinson, C.H. (1997). Diagnostic criteria for complicated grief disorder. *American Journal of Psychiatry, 154*, 904-910.

Hosay, C.K. (2003). The need to educate nursing home administrators about variations in state legislation affecting patients' rights to refuse treatment. *Illness, Crisis & Loss, 11*, 148-161.

Hughes, D. & Kleespies, P. (2001). Suicide in the medically ill. *Suicide and Life-Threatening Behavior, 31* (supplement), 48-59.

Ingham, J.M. & Foley, K.M. (1998). Pain and the barriers to its relief at the end of life: A lesson for improving end-of-life health care. *The Hospice Journal 13*, (1/2) 89 -100.

Ingram, K.M., Jones, D.A., & Smith, N.G. (2001). Adjustment among people who have experienced AIDS-related multiple loss: The role of unsupportive social interactions, social support, and coping. *Omega, 43*, 287-309.

Insurance Institute for Highway Safety. (2003). Q&A teenagers: Underage drinking. Arlington (VA): The Institute. Retrieved on March 11, 2004, from www.iihs.org/safety_facts/qanda/underage.htm

Iserson, K.V. (1999). *Grave words: Notifying survivors about sudden, unexpected deaths.* Tucson, AZ: Galen Press.

Jacobs, S. (1999). *Traumatic grief: Diagnosis, treatment, and prevention.* New York: Brunner/Mazel.

Jacobs, D.G., Brewer, M., & Klein-Benheim, M. (1999). Chapter 1: Suicide Assessment. *The Harvard Medical School guide to suicide assessment and intervention.* San Francisco: Jossey-Bass.

Jacobs, S., Mazure, C., & Prigerson, H. (2000). Diagnostic criteria for traumatic grief. *Death Studies, 24*(3), 185-199.

Jevne, R.F. & Reilly-Williams, D. (1998). *When dreams don't work.* New York: Baywood.

Jones, K. (2001). Last touch. *Nursing2001, 31*(10), 45.

Jordan, J.R. (2001). Is suicide bereavement different? A reassessment of the literature. *Suicide and Life-Threatening Behavior, 31*, 91-102.

Kalish, R.A., (1985). *Death, grief, and caring relationships* (2nd ed.). Monterey, CA: Brooks/Cole.

Kamm, S. & Vandenberg, B. (2001). Grief communication, grief reactions, and marital satisfaction in bereaved parents. *Death Studies, 25*, 569-582.

Kanel, K., (2003). *A guide to crisis intervention* (2nd ed.). Monterey, CA: Brooks/Cole.

Kaplan, L.J. (2000). Toward a model of caregiver grief: Nurses' experiences of treating dying children. *Omega, 41*, 187-206.

Kastenbaum, R. (1999). The moment of death: Is hospice making a difference? *The Hospice Journal, 14*(3/4), 253-270.

Kastenbaum, R. J. (2001). *Death, society, and human experience* (7th ed.). Boston: Allyn and Bacon.

Kavanaugh, K. & Paton, J.B. (2001). Communicating with parents who experience a perinatal loss. *Illness, Crisis & Loss, 9*, 369-380.

Kaye, L.W. & Davitt, J.K. (1998). Comparison of the high-tech service delivery experiences of hospice and non-hospice home health providers. *The Hospice Journal, 13*(3), 1-20.

Kelly, V.L. (2001). The cycle of loss, grief, and violence as exhibited in the lives of inner-city youth. *Illness, Crisis & Loss, 9*, 284-297.

Kenyon, B.L. (2001). Current research in children's conceptions of death: A critical review. *Omega, 43*, 63-91.

Kessler D. (1998). *The rights of the dying.* New York: HarperPerennial.

Klass, D., Silverman, P.S., & Nickman, S.L. (1996). *Continuing bonds: New understanding of grief.* Washington, DC: Taylor & Francis.

Klepac-Lockhart, L., Bookwala. J., Fagerlin, A., Coppola, K.M., Ditto, P.H., Danks, J.H., & Smucker, W.D. (2001). Older adults' attitudes toward death: Links to perceptions of health and concerns about end-of-life issues. *Omega, 43,* 331-347.

Knight, K.H., Elfenbein, M.H., & Capozzi, L. (2000). Relationship of recollections of first death experience to current death attitudes. *Death Studies, 24,* 201-221.

Kubler-Ross, E. (1969). *On death and dying.* New York: MacMillan.

Kunkel, A.D. & Dennis, M.R. (2003). Grief consolation in eulogy rhetoric: An integrative framework. *Death Studies, 27,* 1-38.

Lane, D. (1992). Music therapy: A gift beyond measure. *Oncology Nursing Forum, 19*(6): 863-867.

Lang, A., Goulet, C., Aita, M., Giguere, V., Lamarre, H., & Perreault, E. (2001). Weathering the storm of perinatal bereavement via hardiness. *Death Studies, 25,* 497-512.

Larson, D.G. (1993). *The helper's journey.* Champaign, IL: Research Press

Last Acts. (n.d.) *A vision for better care at the end of life.* Retrieved March 17, 2004, from http://www.lastacts.org/docs/publicprecepts.pdf

Last Acts. (1997). Precepts of palliative care. Retrieved October 11, 2004 from http://www.lastacts.org/docs/profprecepts.pdf

Last Acts, Task Force on Palliative Care. (2001). Care for the spirit: The role of spirituality in end-of-life care. Retrieved October 11, 2004 from http://www.lastacts.org/files/misc/careforspirit.pdf

Lattanzi-Licht, M. & Doka, K.J. (2003). *Living with grief: Coping with public tragedy.* Washington, D.C.: Hospice Foundation of America.

Last Acts. (2001). Care for the spirit. Retrieved August 9, 2003, from http://www.lastacts.org/files/misc/careforspirit.pdf

Lee, R.L.M. (2003). The new face of death: Postmodernity and changing perspectives of the afterlife. *Illness, Crisis & Loss, 11*, 134-147.

Leenaars, A.A. & Wenckstern, S. (1998). Principles of postvention: Applications to suicide and trauma in schools. *Death Studies, 22,* 357-391.

Leichtentritt, R.D. & Rettig, K.D. (2000). The good death: Reaching an inductive understanding. *Omega, 41,* 221-248.

Lester, D., Aldridge, M., Aspenberg, C., Boyle, K., Radsniak, P., & Waldron, C. (2001-2002). What is the afterlife like? Undergraduate beliefs about the afterlife. *Omega, 44,* 113-126.

Lester, D. (1999). The social causes of suicide: A look at Durkheim's *Le Suicide* one hundred years later. *Omega, 40,* 307-321.

Lester, D. & Leenaars, A. (1996). The ethics of suicide and suicide prevention. *Death Studies 20,* 163-184.

Levetown, M., Hayslip, B., & Peel, J. (1999). The development of the physicians' end-of-life care attitude scale. *Omega, 40*(2) 323-333.

Lieberman, M.A. (1997). Bereavement self-help groups: A review of conceptual and methodological issues. In M.S. Stroebe, W. Stroebe, & R.O. Hansson (Eds.), *Handbook of bereavement: Theory, research, and intervention* (pp. 411-426). New York: Cambridge University Press.

Lohan, J.A. & Murphy, S.A. (2001-2002). Parents' perceptions of adolescent sibling grief responses after an adolescent or young adult child's sudden violent death. *Omega, 44,* 195-213.

Lohan, J.A., & Murphy, S.A. (2002). Exploring family functioning after the violent death of a child. *Journal of Family Nursing, 8,* 32-49.

Lund, D.A. & Caserta, N.S. (2002). Facing life alone: Loss of a significant other in later life. In K.J. Doka (Ed.), *Living with grief: Loss in later life* (p.207-224). Washington, D.C.: Hospice Foundation of America.

Madara, E.J. (1999). From church basements to World Wide Web sites: The growth of self-help support groups online. *International Journal of Self-Help and Self-Care, 1*(1), 37-48.

Mak, M.H.J. (2001). Awareness of dying: An awareness of Chinese patients with terminal cancer. *Omega, 43,* 259-279.

Marion, M.S. & Range, L.M. (2003). African-American college women's suicide buffers. *Suicide and Life-Threatening Behavior, 33,* 33-43.

Martin, G. (1998). Media influence to suicide: The search for solutions. *Archives of Suicide Research, 4,* (1), 51-66.

Martin, T.L. & Doka, K.J. (1999). *Men don't cry, women do: Transcending gender stereotypes of grief.* Philadelphia: Brunner/Mazel.

Martin, D.S. & Youngren, K.B. (2000). The virtual community: Helping patients use Internet support groups. *Home Healthcare Nurse, 18*(5), 333-336.

Martinson, I.M. (2001). Barriers and facilitators experienced during my career: From the perspective of being a woman in the field of thanatology. *Illness, Crisis & Loss, 9,* 63-69.

Marwit, S.J. & Datson, S.L. (2002). Disclosure preferences about terminal illness: An examination of decision-related factors. *Death Studies, 26,* 1-20.

Mastrogianis, L. & Lumley, M.A. (2002). Aftercare services from funeral directors to bereaved men: Surveys of both providers and recipients. *Omega, 45,* 167-185.

McBee-Strayer, S. & Rogers, J. (2002). Lesbian, gay, and bisexual suicidal behavior: Testing a constructivist model. *Suicide and Life-Threatening Behavior, 32,* 272-283.

McConnell, E.A. (2001). Myths & facts about communicating clearly. *Nursing2001, 31*(4), 74.

McDaniel, J.S., Purcell, D., & D'Augelli, R. (2001). The relationship between sexual orientation and risk for suicide: Research findings and future directions for research and prevention. *Suicide and Life-Threatening Behavior, 31,* (supplement). 84-105.

McIntosh, J.L. (1993). *USA suicide: 1990 official final data.* Denver: American Association of Suicidology.

Mesler, M.A. & Miller, P.J. (2000). Hospice and assisted suicide: The structure and process of an inherent dilemma. *Death Studies, 24,* 135-155.

Mickley, J.R., Pargament, K.I., Brant, C.R. & Hipp, K.M. (1998). God and the search for meaning among hospice caregivers. *The Hospice Journal, 13*(4), 1-17.

Miller, J. S., Segal, D.L., & Coolidge, F. L. (2001). A comparison of suicidal thinking and reasons for living among younger and older adults. *Death Studies, 25,* 357-365.

Murphy, L.D. (2001). The child left behind, *Nursing2001, 31*(1), 62-63.

Murphy, S.A. (2000). The use of research findings in bereavement programs: A case study. *Death Studies, 24*, 585-602.

Murphy, S.A., Clark-Johnson, L., & Lohan, J. (2003). Finding meaning in a child's violent death: A five-year prospective analysis of parents' personal narratives. *Death Studies, 27*, 381-404.

Murphy, S.A., Johnson. L.C., & Weber, N.A. (2002). Coping strategies following a child's violent death: How parents differ in their responses. *Omega, 45*, 99-118.

Myers, S.S. & Range, L.M. (2002). No-suicide agreements: High school students' perspectives. *Death Studies, 26*, 851-857.

National Center for Health Statistics. (2003a). Home health and hospice care. Hyattsville, MD: CDC. Retrieved October 11, 2003 from http://www.cdc.gov/nchs/fastats/homehosp.htm

National Center for Health Statistics. (2003b). Firearm Mortality. Retrieved January 6, 2003 from http://www.cdc.gov/nchs/fastats/firearms.htm

National Center for HIV, STD and TB Prevention. (2003). *Basic Statistics.* Retrieved on March 17, 2004, from http://www.cdc.gov/hiv/stats.htm#cumaids

National Center for Injury Prevention and Control. (2004). *Teen Drivers.* Retrieved January 6, 2004 from http://www.cdc.gov/ncipc/factsheets/teen-mvh.htm

National Institute of Mental Health (NIMH). (1999). Fact sheet: Depression research at the NIMH. Publication No. 00-4501. Reprinted 2000, updated 2002. Bethesda, MD: NIH.

National Institute of Mental Health. (2003). Men and depression. In *Real Men, Real Depression* campaign. NIH Publication No. 03-4972. Retrieved August 8, 2003 from http://menanddepression.nimh.nih.gov/infopage.asp?id=10#

National Organization of Parents of Murdered Children, Inc. *Proper Death Notification.* Retrieved October 14, 2003 from http://www.pomc.com/survivor.cfm#10

National Organization of Parents Of Murdered Children, Inc. *Information for doctors and nurses.* Retrieved October 14, 2003 from http://www.pomc.com/doctors.cfm

National Organization for Victim Assistance. *For Victims and Survivors.* Retrieved on March 11, 2004, from http://www.trynova.org/for_victims_survivors.html

National Safety Council. (2003). Report on Injuries in America, 2001. Retrieved August 8, 2003 from http://www.nsc.org/library/rept2000.htm

Neimeyer, R.A. (2000). *Lessons of loss: A guide to coping.* Keystone Heights, FL: Psycho-Educational Resources.

Neimeyer, R.A., Fortner, B., & Melby, D. (2001). Personal and professional factors and suicide intervention skills. *Suicide and Life-Threatening Behavior, 31*, 71-82.

Nolen-Hoeksema, S., Larson, J. & Bishop, M. (2000). Predictors of family members' satisfaction with hospice. *The Hospice Journal, 15*(2), 29-48.

Norlander, L. & McSteen, K. (2000). The kitchen table discussion: A creative way to discuss end-of-life issues. *Home Health Nurse, 18*(8), 532-539.

O'Callaghan, C.C. (1996). Complementary therapies in terminal care: Pain, music creativity and music therapy in palliative care. *The American Journal of Hospice & Palliative Care, 2*, 43-49.

O'Connor, M.F. (2002-2003). Making meaning of life events: Theory, evidence, and research directions for an alternative model. *Omega, 46*, 51-75.

O'Connor, S., Deeks, J.J., Hawton, K., Simkin, S., Keen, A., Altman, D.G., et al. (1999). Effects of a drug overdose in a television drama on presentation to hospital for self-poisoning: Time series and questionnaire study. *British Medical Journal, 318*(7189), 972-977.

Olvera, R.L. (2001). Suicidal ideation in Hispanic and mixed ancestry adolescents. *Suicide and Life-Threatening Behavior, 31,* 416-427.

Orbach, I., Stein, D., Shani-Sela, M., & Har-Even, D. (2001). Body attitudes and body experiences in suicidal adolescents. *Suicide and Life-Threatening Behavior, 31,* 237-249.

Ott, C.H. & Lueger, R.J. (2002). Patterns of change in mental health status during the first two years of spousal bereavement. *Death Studies, 26,* 387-411.

Owen, J.E., Goode, K.T., & Haley, W.E. (2001). End-of-life care and reactions to death in African-American and white family caregivers of relatives with Alzheimer's disease. *Omega, 43,* 349-361.

Papadatou, D. (2000). A proposed model of health professional's grieving process. *Omega, 41,* 59-77.

Papadatou, D., Papazoglou, I., Bellali, T., & Petraki, D. (2002). Greek nurse and physician grief as a result of caring for children dying of cancer. *Pediatric Nursing, 28*(4), 345-353.

Parker-Oliver, D. (1999-2000). The social construction of the "dying role" and the hospice drama. *Omega, 40,* 493-512.

Parkes, C.M. (1980). Bereavement counseling; Does it work? BMJ 1980; 281, 3-10.

Parkes, C.M. (2003). Acquainted with grief. *Illness, Crisis & Loss, 11,* 37-46.

Paulozzi, L.J., Saltzman, L.E., Thompson, M.P., & Holmgreen, P. (n.d.). *Surveillance for homicide among intimate partners — United States, 1981-1998.* CDC Surveillance Summaries. October 12, 2001. 50 (SS03);1-16. Retrieved August 9, 2003 from http://www.cdc.gov/mmwr/preview/mmwrhtml/ss5003a1.htm

Pearson, J.L. (2000-2001). Preventing late life suicide: National Institutes of Health initiatives, *Omega, 41,* 9-20.

Peterson, E.M., Luoma, J.B., & Dunne, E. (2002). Suicide survivors' perceptions of the treating clinician. *Suicide and Life-Threatening Behavior, 32,* 158-166.

Pfaadt, M.J. (2000). A review of the basics: Understanding the categories of skilled nursing services. *Home Healthcare Nurse, 18,* (5), 297-300.

Phillips, D.P. (1979). Suicide, motor vehicle fatalities, and the mass media: Evidence toward theory of suggestion. *American Journal of Sociology, 84,* 1150-1174.

Pickett, M., Barg, F.K., & Lynch, M.P. (2001). Development of a home-based family caregiver cancer education program. *The Hospice Journal, 15*(4), 19-40.

Picton, C., Cooper, B.K., Close, D., & Tobin, J. (2001). Bereavement support groups: Timing of participation and reasons for joining. *Omega, 43,* 247-258.

Pollack, C.E. (2003). Intentions of burial: Mourning, politics, and memorials following the massacre at Srebrenica. *Death Studies, 27*(2):125-42, 2003.

Pollock, L.R. & Williams, J.H. (2001). Effective problem solving in suicide attempters depends on specific autobiographical recall. *Suicide and Life-Threatening Behavior, 31*(4), 386-397.

Powell, K.E., Kresnow, M.J., Mercy, J.A., Potter, L.B., Swann, A.C., Frankowski, R.F., et al. (2001). Alcohol consumption and nearly lethal suicide attempts. *Suicide and Life-Threatening Behavior, 32*(1-supplement): 30-41.

Preston, T.A. (1994). *Killing pain, Ending life.* New York Times, November 1, 1994, p. A27.

Prigerson, H., Ahmed, I, Silverman G. K. Saxena, A.T. Maciejewski, P.K. Jacobs, S.C. & Kasal, S.V. (2002). Rates and risks of complicated grief among psychiatric clinic patients in Karachi, Pakistan. *Death Studies, 26*: 781-792.

Prigerson, H.G., Bierhals, A.J., Kasl, S.V., Reynolds, C.F., Shear, M.K., Day, N., et al. (1997). Traumatic grief as a risk factor for mental and physical morbidity. *American Journal of Psychiatry, 54*, 617-623.

Proust, M. (1948). *The maxims of Marcel Proust* (J. O'Brien, Ed. and Trans.). New York City: Columbia University Press. (Original work published 1921.)

Ragow-Obrien, D., Hayslip, B., & Guarnaccia, C.A. (2000). The impact of hospice on attitudes toward funerals and subsequent bereavement adjustment. *Omega, 41*, 291-305.

Rando, T.A. (1984). *Grief, dying, and death: Clinical interventions for caregivers.* Champaign, IL: Research Press.

Rando, T.A. (1992). The increasing prevalence of complicated mourning: The onslaught is just beginning. *Omega, 26*, 43-59.

Rando, T.A. (1993). *Treatment of complicated mourning.* Champaign, IL: Research Press.

Rando, T.A. (2000). *Clinical dimensions of anticipatory mourning.* Champaign, IL: Research Press.

Raphael, B., Middleton, W., Martinek, N., & Misso, V. (1997). Counseling and therapy of the bereaved. In M.S. Stroebe, W. Stroebe, & R.O. Hansson (Eds.), *Handbook of bereavement: Theory, research, and intervention* (pp 427-453). New York: Cambridge University Press.

Reese, D.J. (2000). The role of primary caregiver denial in inpatient placement during home hospice care. *The Hospice Journal, 15*(1), 15-33.

Reid, J.K. & Reid, C.L. (2001). A cross marks the spot: A study of roadside death memorials in Texas and Oklahoma. *Death Studies, 25*, 341-356.

Reilly-Smorawski, B., Armstrong, A.V., & Catlin, E.A. (2002). Bereavement support for couples following death of a baby: Program development and 14-year exit analysis. *Death Studies, 26*, 21-37.

Reinhard, S. (2001). Nursing's role in family caregiver support. In Doka, K.J. & Davidson, J.D. (Eds.), *Caregiving and loss: Family needs, professional responses* (pp. 181-190). Washington, DC: Hospice Foundation of America.

Rich, D. (2000). The impact of postpregnancy loss services on grief outcome: Integrating research and practice in the design of perinatal bereavement programs. *Illness, Crisis & Loss, 8*, 244-264.

Richards, T.A., Wrubel, J., & Folkman, S.. (1999-2000). Death rites in the San Francisco gay community: Cultural developments of the AIDS epidemic. *Omega, 40*, 335-350.

Richardson, V.E. & Balaswamy, S. (2001). Coping with bereavement among elderly widowers. *Omega, 43*, 129-144.

Riches, G. & Dawson, P. (2002). Shoestrings and bricolage: Some notes on researching the impact of a child's death on family relationships. *Death Studies, 26*, 209-222.

Rilke, R.M. (1984). *Letters to a young poet.* New York: Vintage Books.

Ron, P. (2002). Suicidal ideation and depression among institutionalized elderly: The influence of residency duration. *Illness, Crisis & Loss, 10,* 334-343.

Roy, A. (2001). Consumers of mental health services. *Suicide and Life-Threatening Behavior, 31*(supplement), 60-83.

Rubel, B. (1999a). Reducing the risk of suicide ideation by managing pain and treating underlying depression. *Illness, Crisis & Loss, 7,* 325-332.

Rubel, B. (1999b). The grief response experienced by the survivors of suicide. *The Thanatology Newsletter, 6* (1), 8-10.

Rubel, B. (1999c). *But I didn't say goodbye: For parents and professionals helping child suicide survivors.* Kendall Park, NJ: Griefwork Center.

Rubel, B. (1999d). Impact of a grief-crisis intervention immediately after a sudden violent death on the survivor's ability to cope. *Illness, Crisis & Loss, 7,* 376-389.

Rybarik, F. (2000). Perinatal bereavement. *Illness, Crisis & Loss, 8,* 221-226.

Sanders, C. (2001). A woman of many abilities. *Illness, Crisis & Loss, 9,* 50-54.

Sanders, C.M. (1997). Risk factors in bereavement outcome. In M.S. Stroebe, W. Stroebe, & R.O. Hansson (Eds.), *Handbook of bereavement: Theory, research, and intervention* (pp. 255-267). New York: Cambridge University Press.

Scott, S. (2000). Grief reactions to the death of a divorced spouse revisited. *Omega, 41,* 207-219.

Siegel, K. (1986). Psychosocial aspects of rational suicide. *American Journal of Psychotherapy, 40,* 405-418.

Shneidman, E. (1993). *Suicide as psychache: A clinical approach to self-destructive behavior.* Northvale, NJ: Jason Aronson.

Schuchter, S. R. & Zisook, S. (1988). Widowhood: The continuing relationship with the dead spouse. *Bulletin of the Menninger Clinic, 52,* 269-279.

Siebold, C. (1992). *The hospice movement: Easing death's pains.* New York: Twayne.

Silverdale, N. & Katz, J. (2003). Changes in attitudes and practice toward dying people after completion of a U.K.-based distance learning death and dying course. *Illness, Crisis & Loss, 1,* 183-196.

Silverman, P.R. (2001). It makes a difference. *Illness, Crisis & Loss, 9,* 111-128.

Silverman, P.R. & Nickman, S. (1996). Concluding thoughts. In D. Klass, P.R. Silverman, & S. Nickman (Eds.), *Continuing bonds: New understandings of grief* (pp. 349-355). Washington, D.C.: Taylor & Francis.

Silverman, P.R., Nickman, S., & Worden, J.W. (1995). Detachment revisited: The child's reconstruction of a dead parent. In K.J. Doka, (Ed.), *Mourning children, Children mourning* (pp. 131-148). Washington, D.C.: Hospice Foundation of America.

Smith, C.M. (2000). False expectations? Expectations vs. probabilities for dying. *Omega, 41,* 157-185.

Smith, J.C. (2002). *Stress management: A comprehensive handbook of techniques and strategies.* New York: Springer.

Speece, M.W. & Brent, S.B. (1984). Children's understanding of death: A review of three components of a death concept. *Child Development, 55*(5), 1671-1686.

Speece, M.W. & Brent, S.B. (1992). The acquisition of a mature understanding of three components of the concept of death. *Death Studies, 16*(3), 211-229.

Spooren D.J., Henderich, H., & Jannes, C. (2000). Survey description of stress of parents bereaved from a child killed in a traffic accident. A retrospective study of a victim support group. *Omega, 42*(2), 171-185.

Stamm, B.H. (1995). Preface. In B.H. Stamm (Ed.), *Secondary traumatic stress: Self-care issues for clinicians, researchers, and educators* (p. ix-xii). Lutherville, MA: Sidran Press.

Steinhauser, K.E., Maddox, G.L., Person, J.L. & Tulsky, J.A. (2000). The evolution of volunteerism and professional staff within hospice care in North Carolina. *The Hospice Journal, 15*, (1), 35-51.

Stewart, A.E., Lord, J.H., & Mercer, D.L. (2000). A survey of professionals' training and experiences in delivering death notifications. *Death Studies, 24*: 611-631.

Stillion, J.M. & Noviello, S.B. (2001). Living and dying in different worlds: Gender difference in violent death and grief. *Illness, Crisis & Loss, 9*, 247-259.

Straub, S.H. & Roberts, J.M. (2001). Fear of death in widows: Effects of age at widowhood and suddenness of death. *Omega, 43*, 25-41, 2001.

Street, A. & Kissane, D.W. (1999-2000). Dispensing death, desiring death: An exploratory of medical roles and patient motivation during the period of legalized euthanasia in Australia. *Omega, 40*, 231-248.

Stroebe, M. & Schut, H. (1998). Culture and grief. *Bereavement Care, 17*(1), 7-10.

Stroebe, M.S., Stroebe, W. & Hansson, R.O. (Eds.). (1997). *Handbook of bereavement: Theory, research and intervention* (p. 3-19). New York: Cambridge University Press.

Stuart, B. (1999). The NHO medical guidelines for non-cancer disease and local medical review policy: Hospice access for patients with diseases other than cancer. *The Hospice Journal, 14*(3/4), 139-154.

Stuart, C., Waalen, J.K., & Haelstromm, E. (2003). Many helping hearts: An evaluation of peer gatekeeper training in suicide risk assessment. *Death Studies, 27*, 321-333.

Stylianos, S.K. & Vachon, M.L. (1997). The role of social support in bereavement. In M.S. Stroebe, W. Stroebe, & R.O. Hansson (Eds.), *Handbook of bereavement: Theory, research, and intervention* (pp. 397-410). New York: Cambridge University Press.

Templer, D.I., Harville, M., Hutton, S., Underwood, R., Tomeo, M., Russell, M., et al. (2001-2002). Death depression scale—revised. *Omega, 44*, 105-112.

Testimony of Dr. Kathleen M. Foley, Senate Committee on the Judiciary, Hearing entitled, "H.R. 2260, Pain Relief Promotion Act," April 25, 2000. Retrieved August 9, 2003, from http://www.senate.gov/~judiciary/oldsite/42520kf.htm.

Thomson, J.E. (2000). The place of spiritual well-being in hospice patients' overall quality of life. *The Hospice Journal, 15*(2), 13-27.

Tyson-Rawson, K.J. (1997). Adolescent responses to the death of a parent. In C.A. Corr & D.E. Balk (Eds.), *Handbook of adolescent death and bereavement* (pp. 312-328). New York: Springer.

Ufema, J. (2002). Listening: Running out of time? *Nursing 2002, 32*(7), 24.

Ujda, R.M. & Bendiksen, R. (2000). Health care provider support and grief after a perinatal loss: A qualitative study. *Illness, Crisis & Loss, 8*, 265-285.

United Network for Organ Sharing. Retrieved October 11, 2003 from http://www.unos.org.

Uren, T.H. & Wastell, C.A. (2002). Attachment and meaning-making in perinatal bereavement. *Death Studies, 26*, 279-308.

U.S. Bureau of the Census. (1999). Statistical abstract of the United States: Table 140, Deaths by age and leading causes of deaths in 1996 (p. 102). Washington, D.C.: U.S. Government Printing Office. Retrieved August 10, 2003, from http://www.census.gov/prod/99pubs/99statab/sec02.pdf

U.S. Department of Health and Human Services. (2001). *Grief and emotional response advice.* Washington, D.C.: HHS Press Office.

U.S. Public Health Service. (1999). *The Surgeon General's call to action to prevent suicide.* Washington, D.C.: Department of Health & Human Services. Retrieved October 7, 2003 from http://www.surgeongeneral.gov/library/calltoaction/calltoaction.htm

Valentine, L. (1997). Professional interventions to assist adolescents who are coping with death and bereavement. In C.A. Corr & D.E. Balk (Eds.), *Handbook of adolescent death and bereavement* (pp. 312-328). New York: Springer.

Van der Kloot Meijburg, H.H. (2000). The lessons we learn: Palliative care in the Netherlands. *Illness, Crisis & Loss, 8*, 109-119.

Vickio, C.J. (1999). Together in spirit: Keeping our relationships alive when loved ones die. *Death Studies, 23*, 161-175.

Vickio, C.J. (2000). Developing beliefs that are compatible with death: Revising our assumptions about predictability, control, and continuity. *Death Studies, 24*, 739-758.

Walsh-Burke, K. (2000). Matching bereavement services to level of need. *The Hospice Journal, 15*(1), 77-86.

*Webster's New Collegiate Dictionary.* (1977). MA: G. & C. Merriam Company.

Wee, D. & Myers, D. (2003). Compassion satisfaction, compassion fatigue, and critical incident stress management. *International Journal of Emergency Mental Health, 5*(1), 33-37.

Weisman, A.D. (1972). *On dying and denying: A psychiatric study of terminality.* New York: Behavioral Publications.

Welch, K.J. & Bergen, M.B. (1999-2000). Adolescent parent mourning reactions associated with stillbirth or neonatal death. *Omega, 40*, 435-451.

Werth, J.L. (1996). *Rational suicide?: Implications for mental health professionals.* Washington DC: Taylor and Francis.

Werth, J.L. (1999). The role of the mental health professional in helping significant others of persons who are assisted in death. *Death Studies, 23*, 239-255.

Werth, J.L. (2000). How do the mental health issues differ in the withholding/withdrawing of treatment verses assisted death? *Omega, 41*, 259-278.

Werth, J.L. (2001). Policy and psychosocial considerations associated with non-physician assisted suicide: A commentary on Ogden. *Death Studies, 25*, 403-411.

Wheeler, A.R. & Austin, J. (2000). The loss response list: A tool for measuring adolescent grief responses. *Death Studies, 24*, 21-34.

Wheeler, I. (2001). Parental bereavement: The crisis of meaning. *Death Studies, 25*, 51-66.

Wickie, S.K. & Marwit, S.J. (2000-2001), Assumptive world views and the grief reactions of parents of murdered children. *Omega, 42*, 101-113.

Williams, J., Hackworth, S.R., & Cradock, M.M. (2002). Medical crisis and loss clinic: Novel approach to family transitions. *Illness, Crisis & Loss, 10*, 356-366.

Wittkowski, J., The construction of the multidimensional orientation toward dying and death inventory (MODDI-F). *Death Studies, 25*, 479-495.

Witt-Sherman, D. (1999). End-of-life care: Challenges and opportunities for health care professionals. *The Hospice Journal, 14*(3/4), 109-121.

Wood, J.D. & Milo, E. (2000). Father's grief when a disabled child dies. *Death Studies, 25*, 635-661.

Worden, J.W. (1991). *Grief counseling and grief therapy.* New York: Springer.

Worden, J.W. (2002). *Grief counseling and grief therapy* (3rd ed.). New York: Springer.

Worthen, L.T. & Yeatts, D.E. (2000-2001). Assisted suicide: Factors affecting public attitudes. *Omega, 42*, 115-135.

Yang, S.C. & Chen, S.F. (2002). A phenomenographic approach to the meaning of death: A Chinese perspective. *Death Studies, 26*, 143-175.

Young, M.E. (1997). How to avoid becoming a zombie. In J. Kottler (Ed.), *Finding your way as a counselor* (p. 45-48). Alexandria, VA: American Counseling Association.

Zinner, E.S. (2000). Being a man about it: The marginalization of men in grief. *Illness, Crisis & Loss, 8*, 181-188.

Zuberbueler, E. (1996). Complementary therapies in terminal care, Massage therapy: An added dimension in terminal care. *The American Journal of Hospice & Palliative Care, 13*(2), 50.

Zucker, A. (1995). The right to die. *Death Studies, 19*, 293-298.

# INDEX

# PRETEST KEY

# Death, Dying, and Bereavement:
## Providing Compassion During a Time of Need

| | | |
|---|---|---|
| 1. | d | Chapter 1 |
| 2. | a | Chapter 1 |
| 3. | d | Chapter 1 |
| 4. | a | Chapter 2 |
| 5. | c | Chapter 2 |
| 6. | a | Chapter 3 |
| 7. | d | Chapter 3 |
| 8. | c | Chapter 4 |
| 9. | d | Chapter 5 |
| 10. | d | Chapter 5 |
| 11. | a | Chapter 6 |
| 12. | d | Chapter 6 |
| 13. | c | Chapter 7 |
| 14. | c | Chapter 7 |
| 15. | b | Chapter 7 |
| 16. | d | Chapter 7 |
| 17. | d | Chapter 8 |
| 18. | a | Chapter 8 |
| 19. | c | Chapter 9 |
| 20. | b | Chapter 9 |

# Western Schools® offers over 60 topics to suit all your interests – and requirements!

## Clinical Conditions/Nursing Practice

A Nurse's Guide to Weight Control
for Healthy Living ..............................25 hrs
Auscultation Skills: Breath and Heart Sounds ......12 hrs
Basic Nursing of Head, Chest, Abdominal,
Spine and Orthopedic Trauma ......................16 hrs
Care at the End of Life .................................3 hrs
Chest Tube Management ................................2 hrs
Diabetes Nursing Care ................................30 hrs
Healing Nutrition ......................................24 hrs
Hepatitis C: The Silent Killer ........................2 hrs
HIV/AIDS.........................................1, 2, 4 or 30 hrs
Holistic & Complementary Therapies: Introduction..1 hr
Influenza: A Vaccine-Preventable Disease ................1 hr
Managing Obesity and Eating Disorders ..............30 hrs
Pain Management: Principles and Practice...........30 hrs
Popular Diets and Diet Drugs ........................2 hrs
Practical Weight Control: Assessment & Planning..7 hrs
Practical Weight Control: Lifestyle Interventions..10 hrs
Pressure Ulcers: Guidelines for Prevention
and Nursing Management................................30 hrs
The Neurological Exam...................................1 hr

## Cosmetic Treatments/Surgery

Belt Lipectomy: Lower Body Contouring ................1 hr
Botox Treatments and Dermal Fillers......................1 hr
Cosmetic Breast Surgery ...................................1 hr
Weight Loss Surgery .......................................1 hr

## Critical Care/ER/OR

Ambulatory Surgical Care ............................20 hrs
Case Studies in Critical Care Nursing:
A Guide for Application and Review ..............36 hrs
Principles of Basic Trauma Nursing .....................30 hrs

## Geriatrics

Alzheimer's: Things a Nurse Needs to Know........12 hrs
Elder Abuse ............................................4 hrs
Home Health Nursing ..................................30 hrs
Major Issues in Gerontological Nursing ................10 hrs
Nursing Care of the Older Adult ...........................30 hrs

## Infectious Diseases/Bioterrorism

Biological Weapons ....................................5 hrs
Bioterrorism & the Nurse's Response to WMD ......5 hrs
Influenza: A Vaccine-Preventable Disease ................1 hr
SARS: An Emerging Public Health Threat ..............1 hr
Smallpox.................................................2 hrs
The New Threat of Drug Resistant Microbes ..........5 hrs
West Nile Virus ..........................................1 hr

## Maternal-Child/Pediatrics/Women's Health

Attention Deficit Hyperactivity Disorders
Throughout the Lifespan................................30 hrs
Challenges in Women's Health: PMS;
Reproductive Choices; Menopause;
Gynecological Disorders ............................2-5 hrs
End-of-Life Care for Children and
Their Families ......................................2 hrs
IPV (Intimate Partner Violence):
A Domestic Violence Concern ...................1 or 3 hrs
Manual of School Health ..............................30 hrs
Maternal-Newborn Nursing..............................30 hrs
Pediatric Nursing: Routine to Emergent Care........30 hrs
Pediatric Pharmacology ................................10 hrs
Pediatric Physical Assessment.............................10 hrs
Women's Health: Contemporary
Advances and Trends ...............................30 hrs

## Oncology

Cancer in Women.......................................30 hrs
Cancer Nursing: A Solid Foundation for Practice ..30 hrs
Chemotherapy Essentials: Principles & Practice ..15 hrs

## Professional Issues/Management/Law

Medical Error Prevention: Patient Safety ................2 hrs
Nursing Ethics and the Law...............................30 hrs
Nursing and Malpractice Risks:
Understanding the Law .............................30 hrs
Ohio Law: Standards of Safe Nursing Practice ........1 hr
Supervisory Skills for Nurses ..........................30 hrs
Surviving and Thriving in Nursing ......................30 hrs
Understanding Managed Care ...............................30 hrs

## Psychiatric/Mental Health

Basic Psychopharmacology...............................5 hrs
Child Abuse .............................................30 hrs
IPV (Intimate Partner Violence):
A Domestic Violence Concern ...................1 or 3 hrs
Psychiatric Principles & Applications for
General Patient Care ...............................30 hrs
Psychiatric Nursing Update: Current Trends
in Diagnosing and Treatment ........................30 hrs
Substance Abuse .......................................30 hrs

**Visit us online at www.westernschools.com for these great courses – plus all the latest CE topics!**
Online testing also available.                                    REV. 3/04 v2